PSALM 23

The LORD is my shepherd;
I shall not want.

He maketh me to lie down in green
pastures: he leadeth me beside
the still waters.

He restoreth my soul: he leadeth me
in the paths of righteousness for
his name's sake.

Yea, though I walk through the valley
of the shadow of death, I will fear no evil:
for thou art with me; thy rod and thy
staff they comfort me.

Thou preparest a table before me in the
presence of mine enemies: thou anointest
my head with oil; my cup runneth over.

Surely goodness and mercy shall follow
me all the days of my life: and I will dwell
in the house of the LORD for ever.

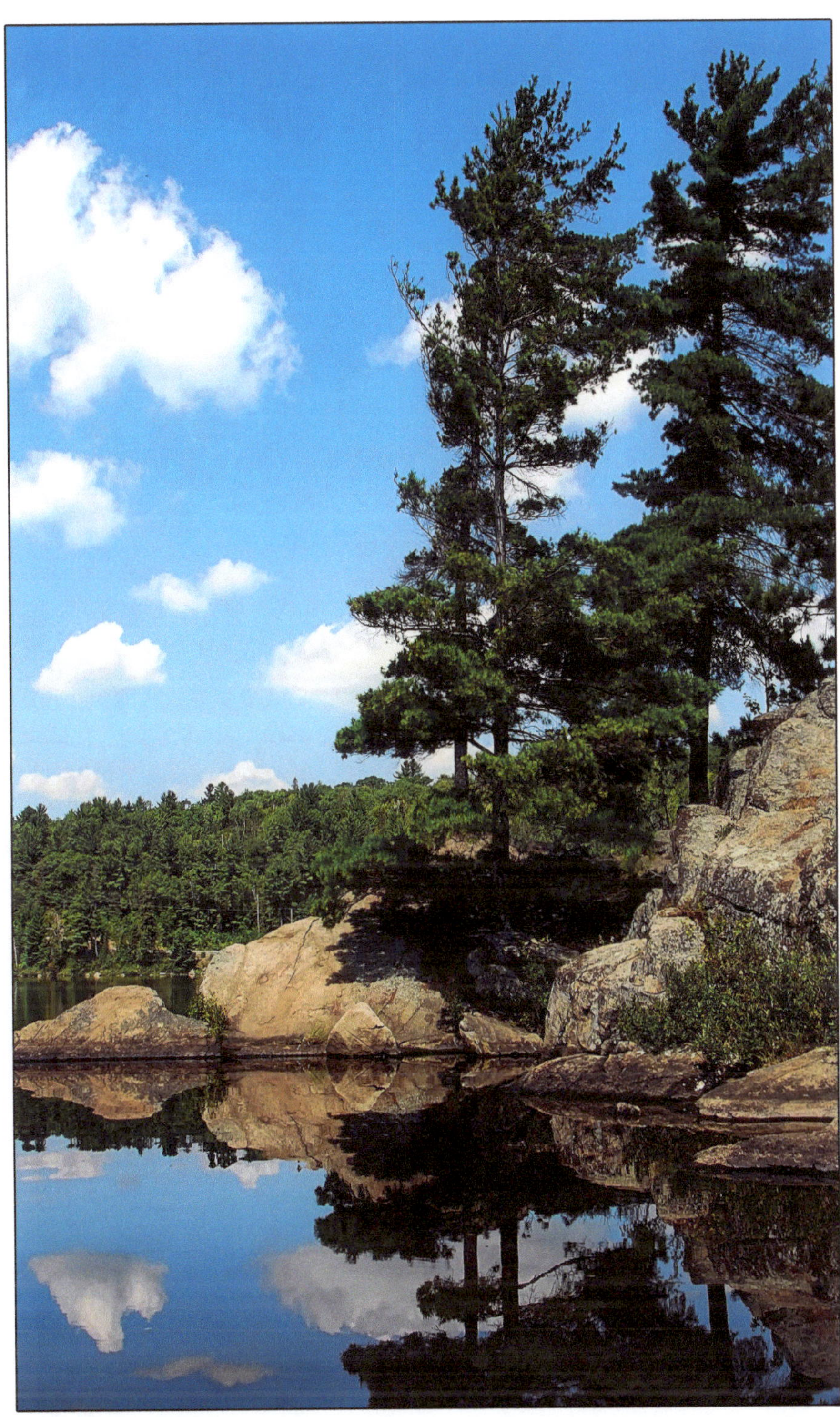

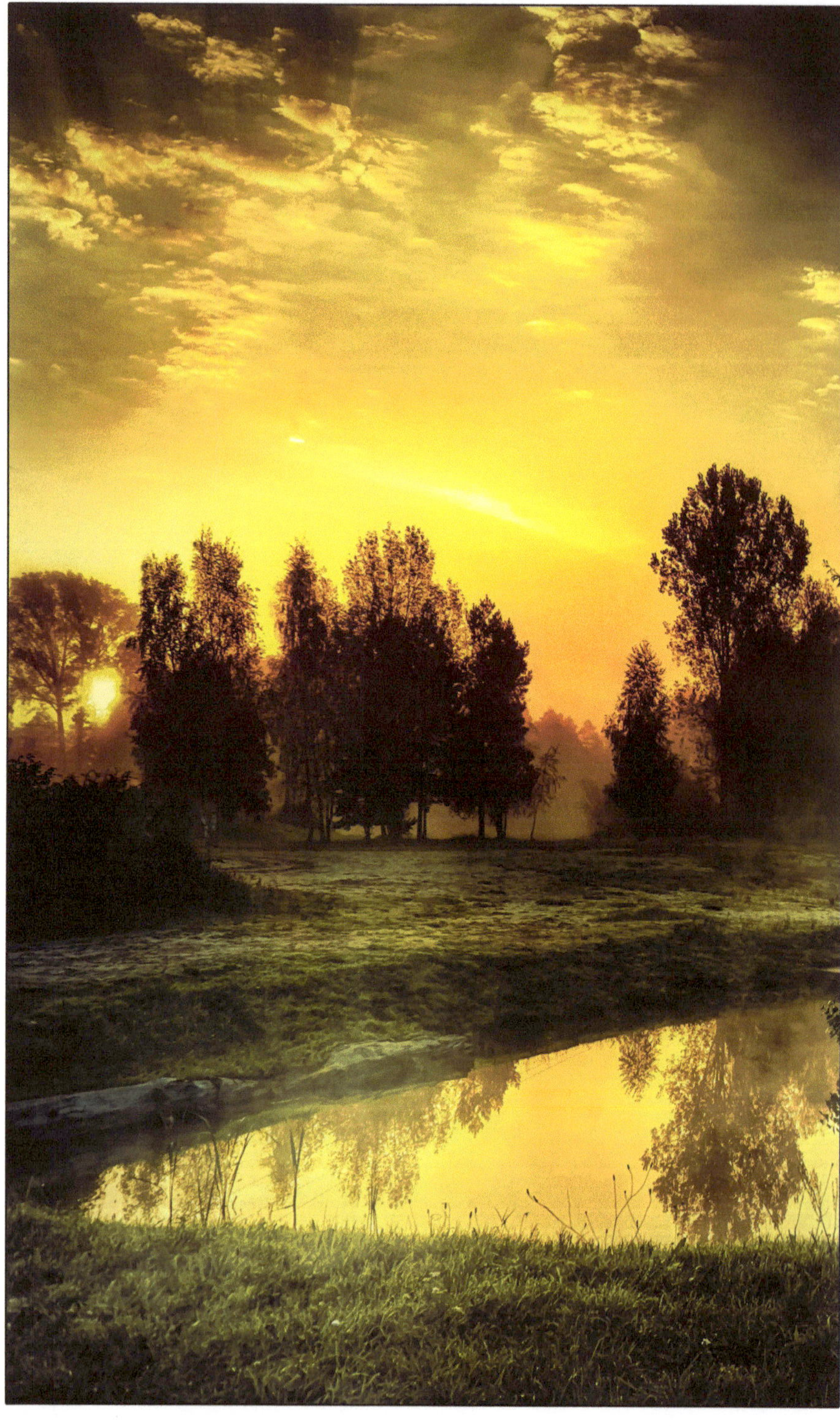

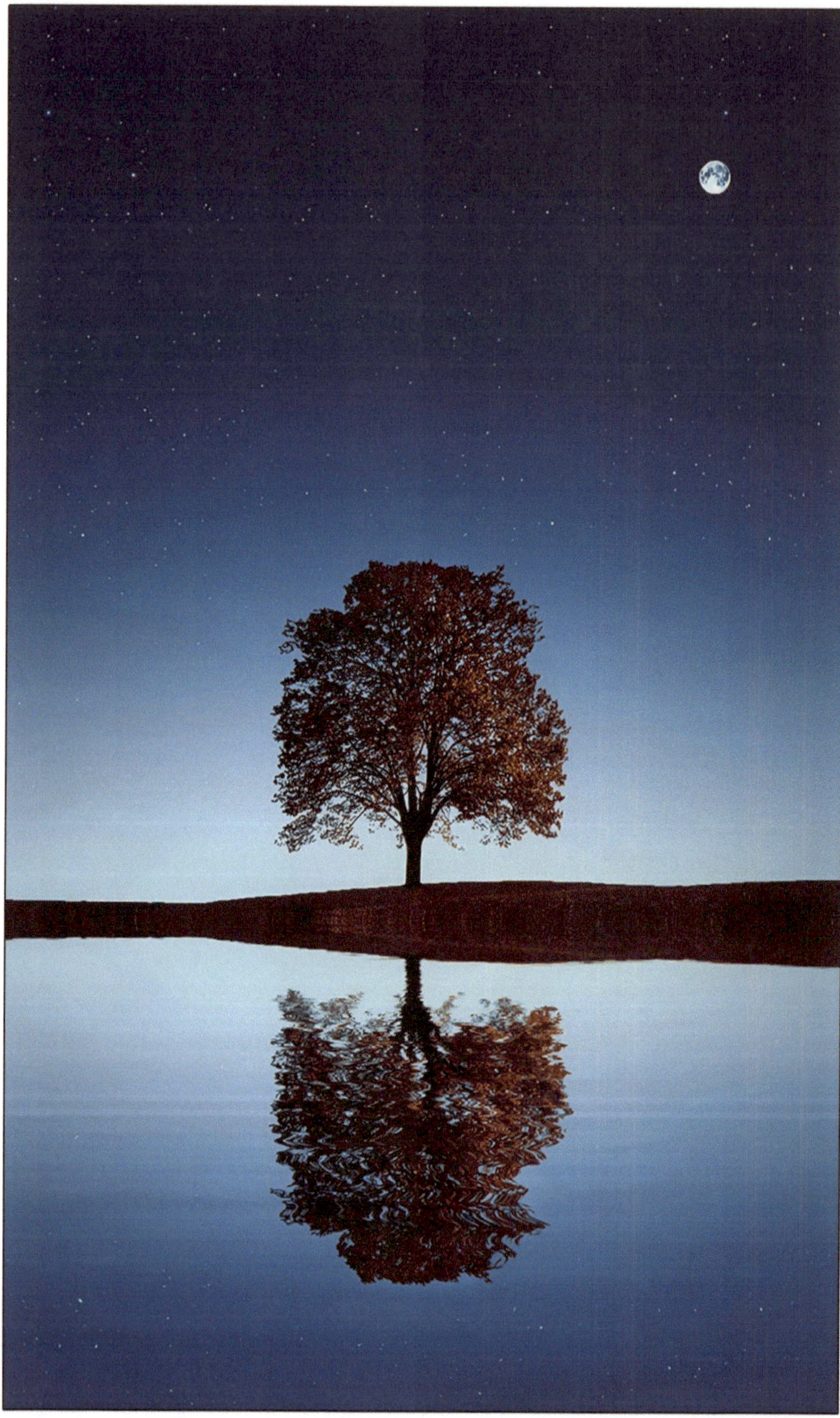

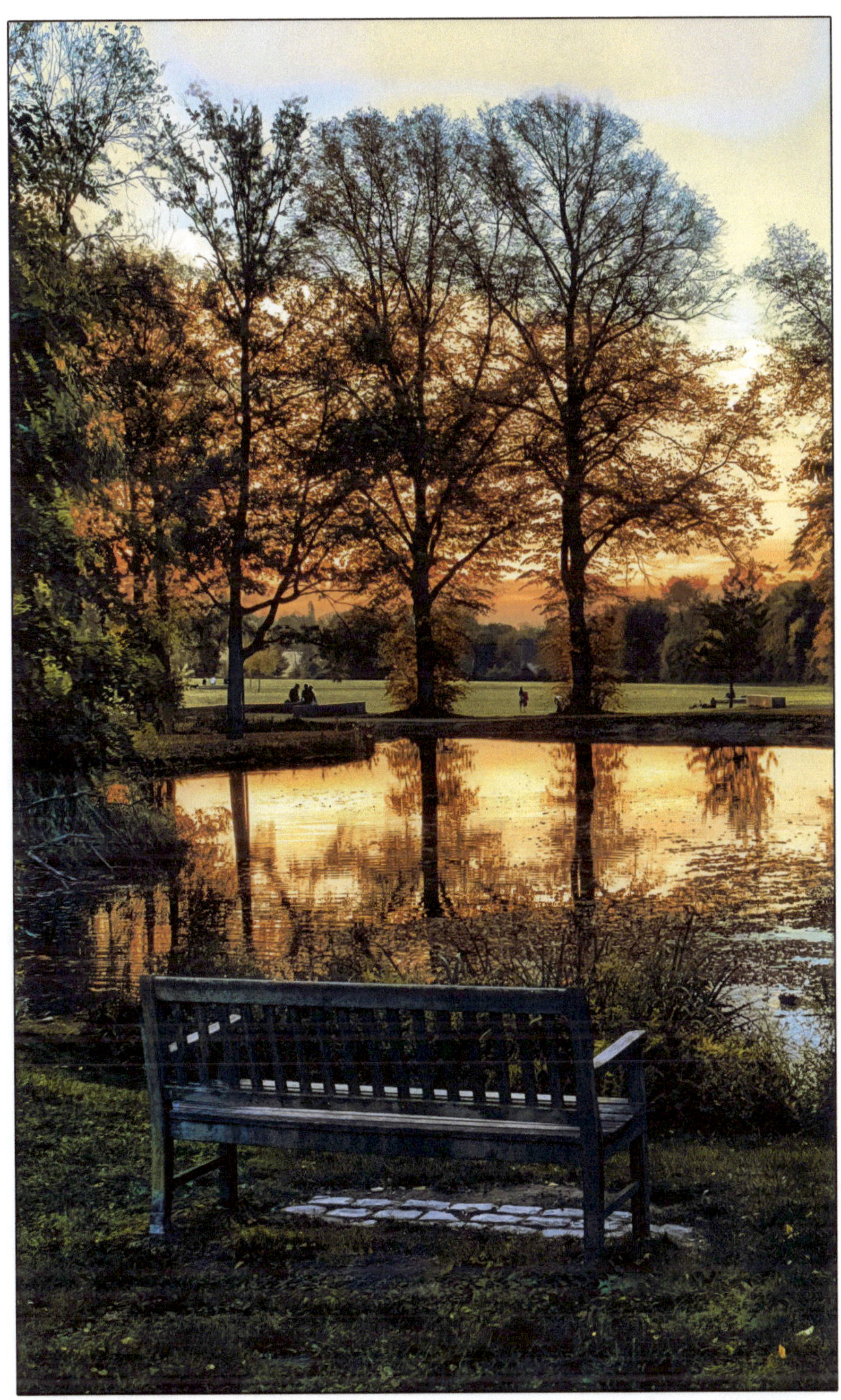

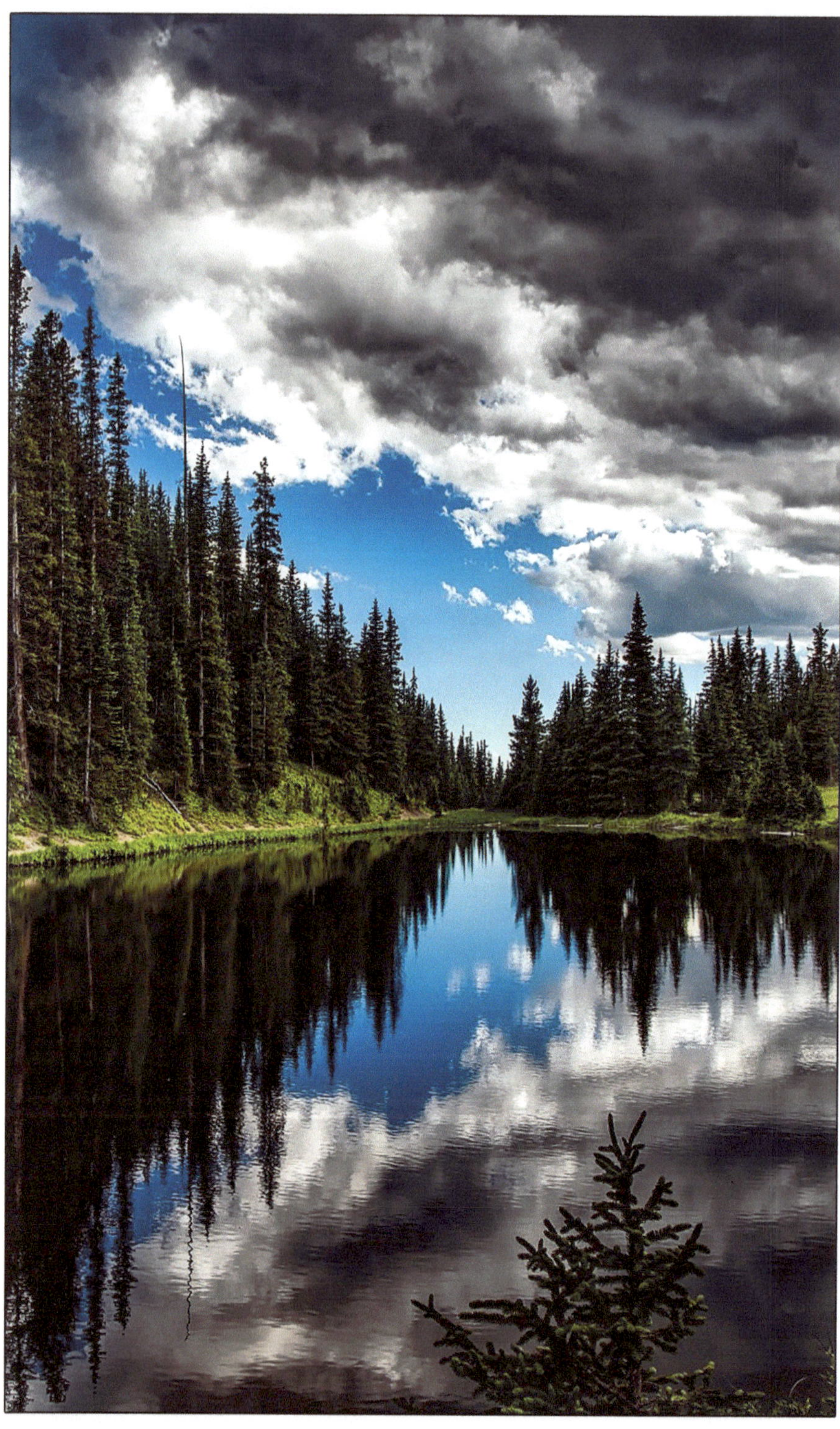

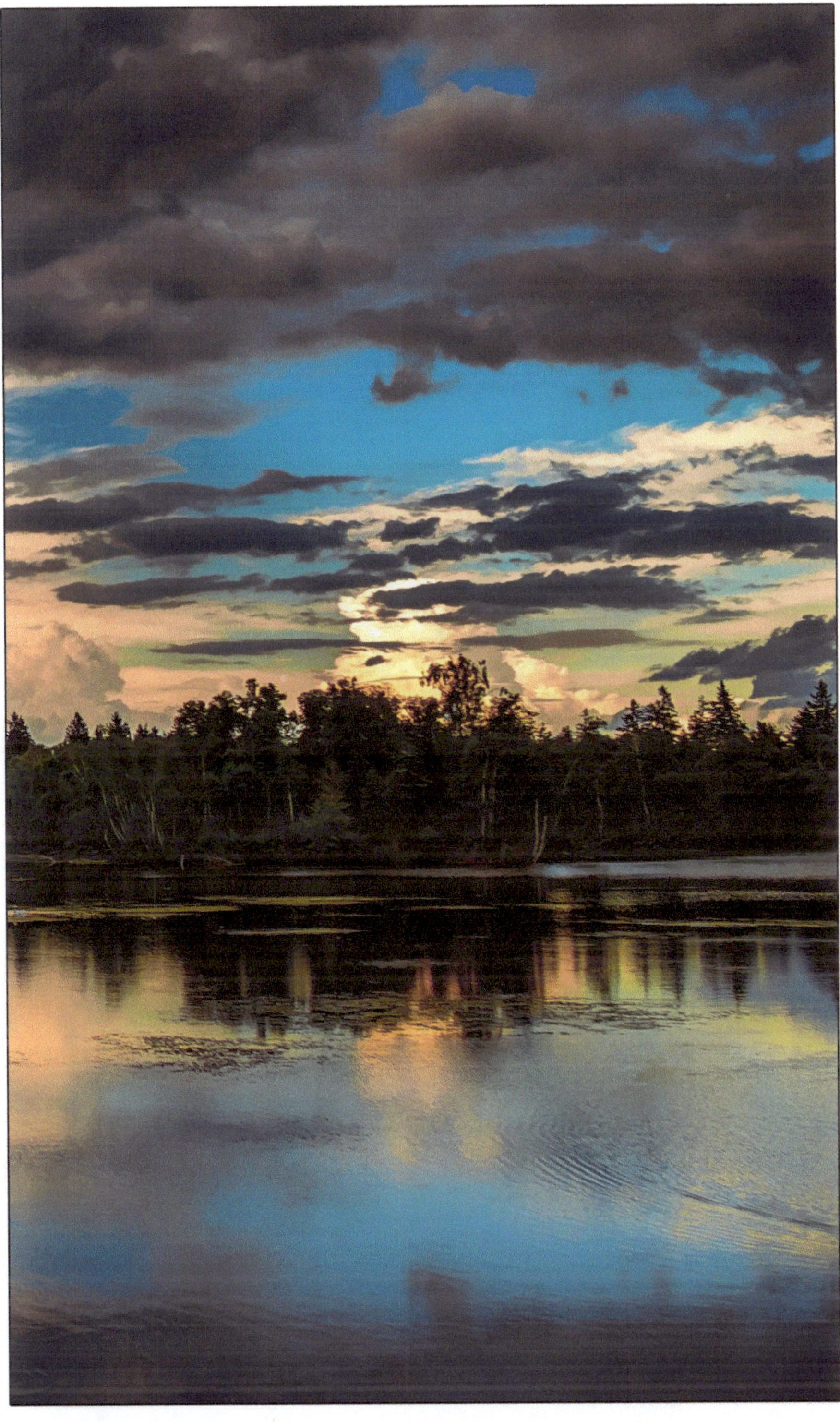

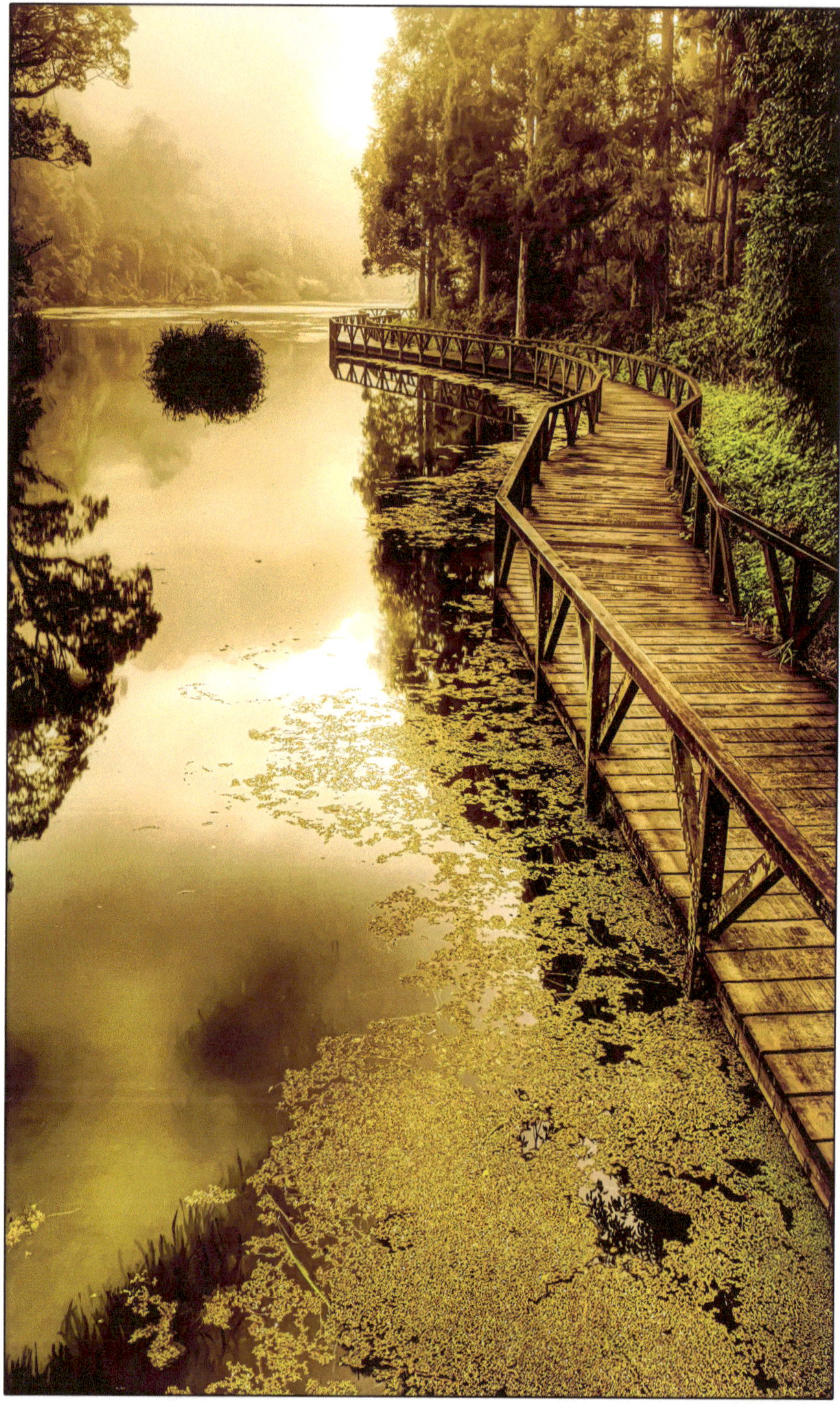

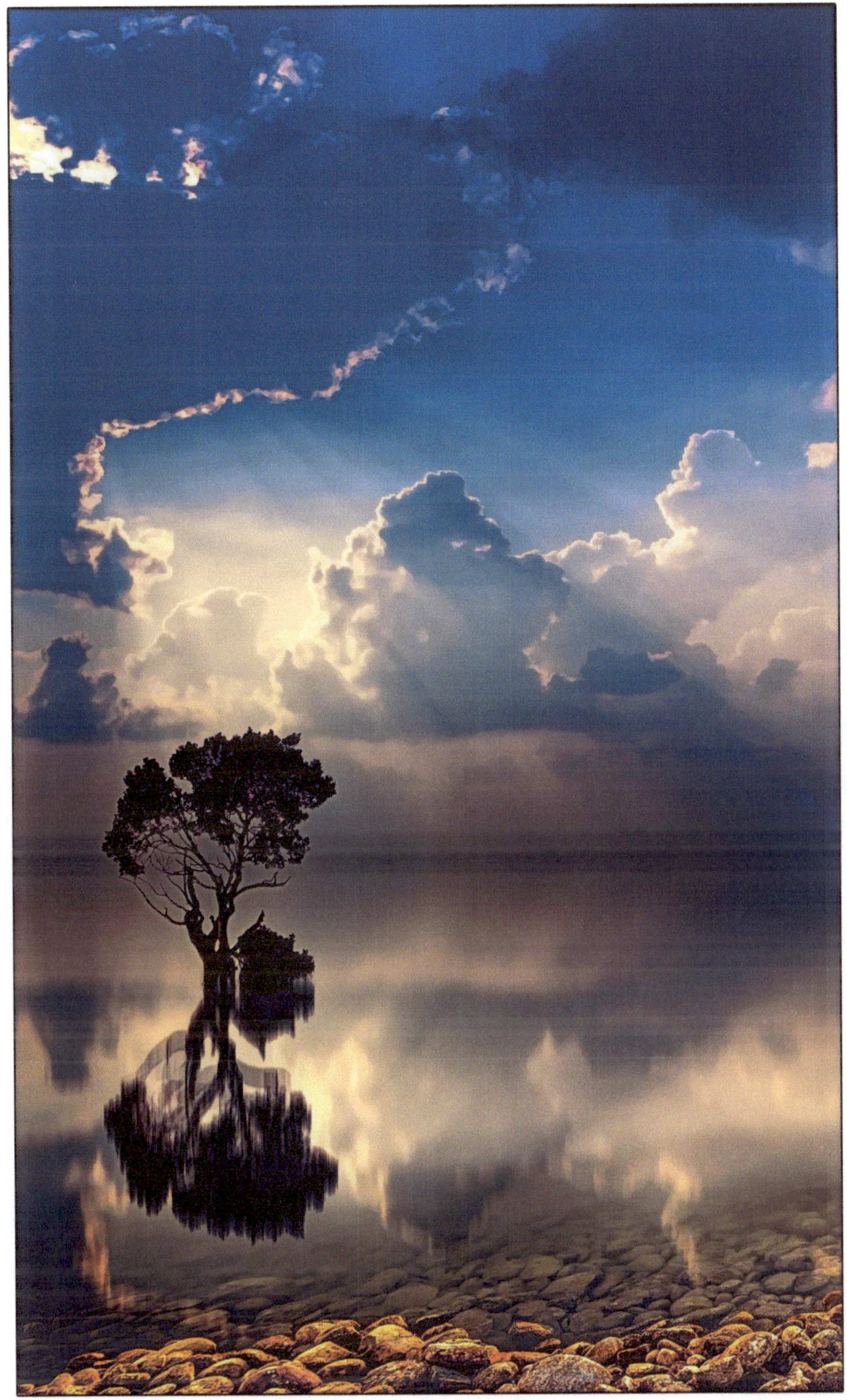

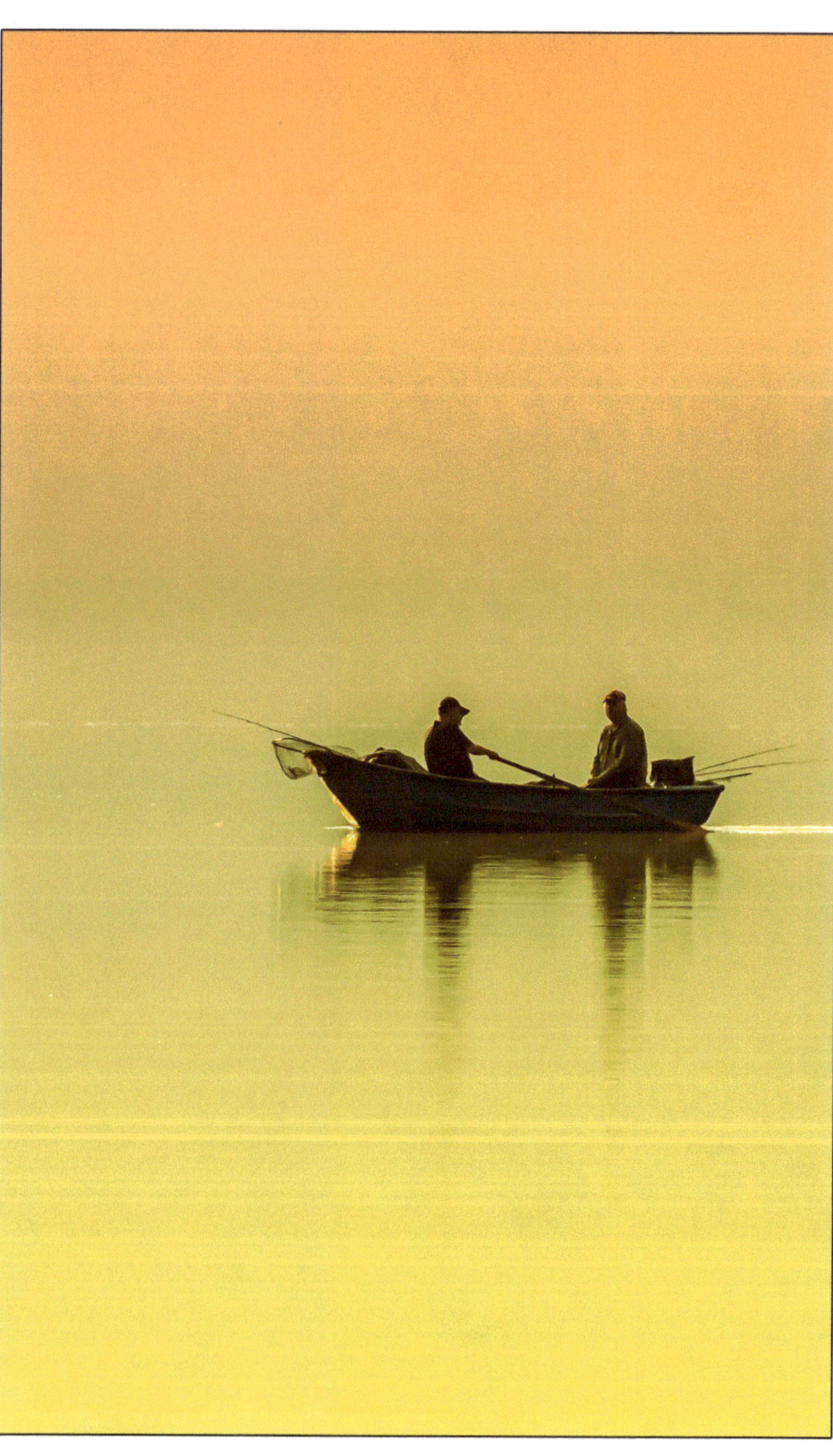

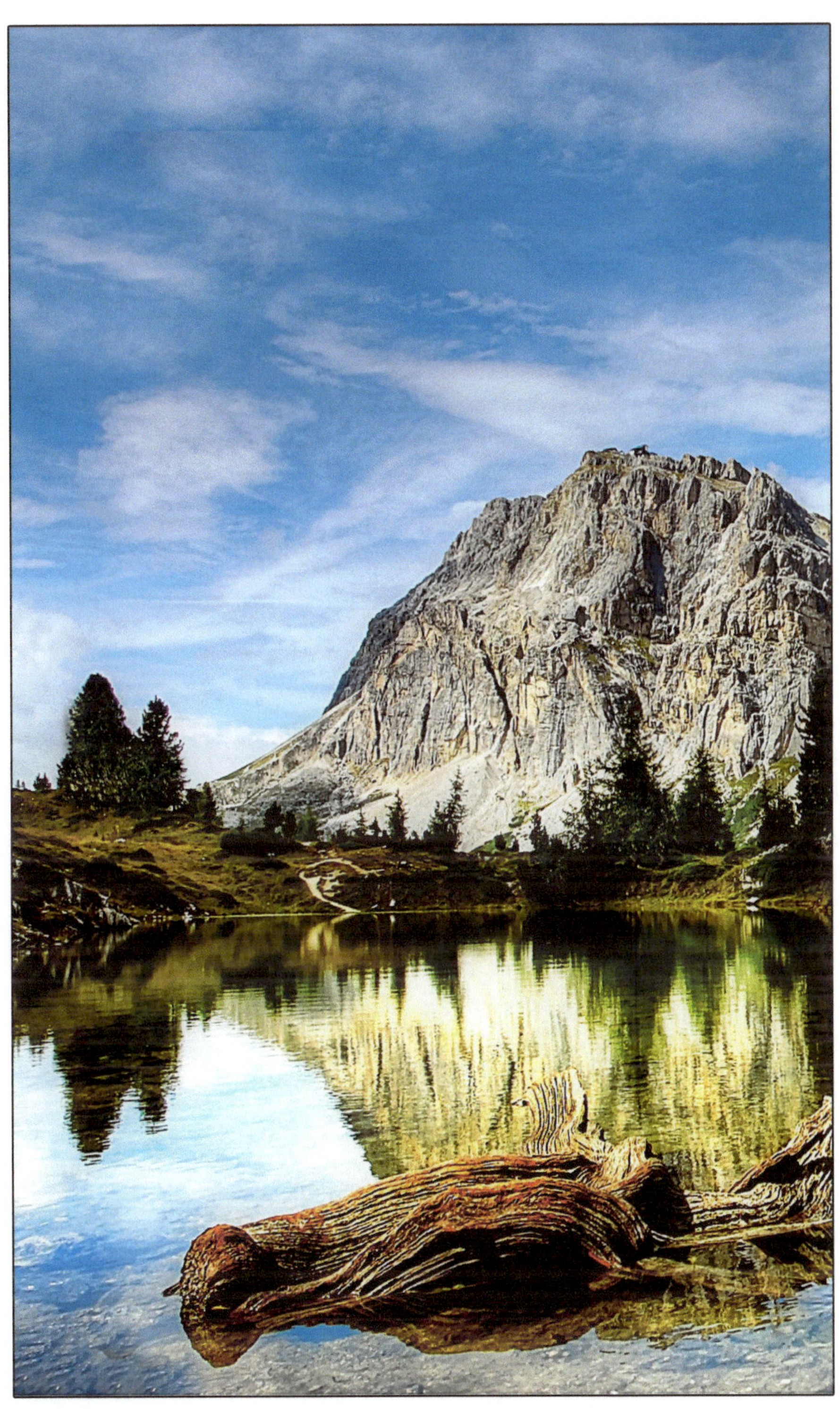

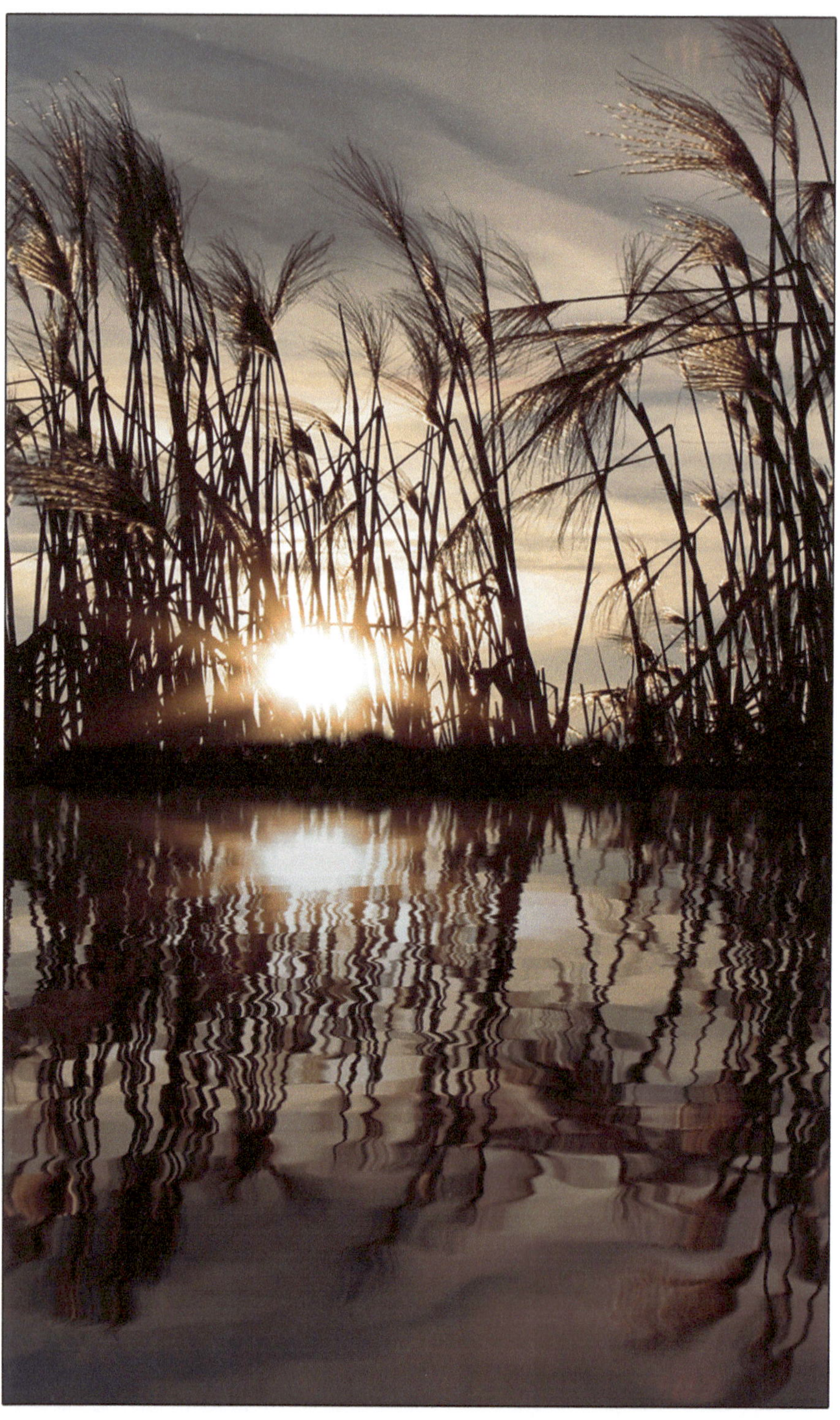

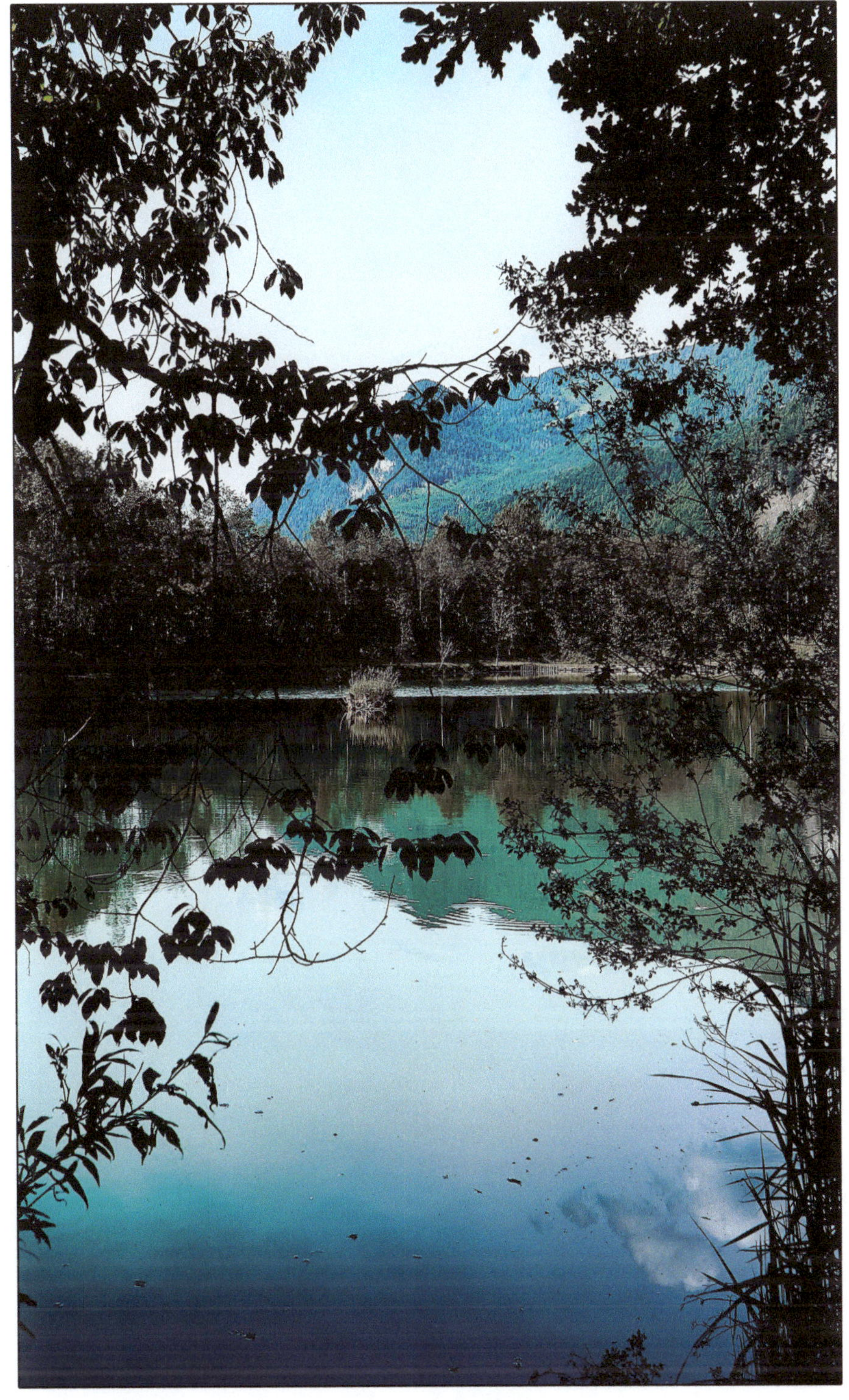

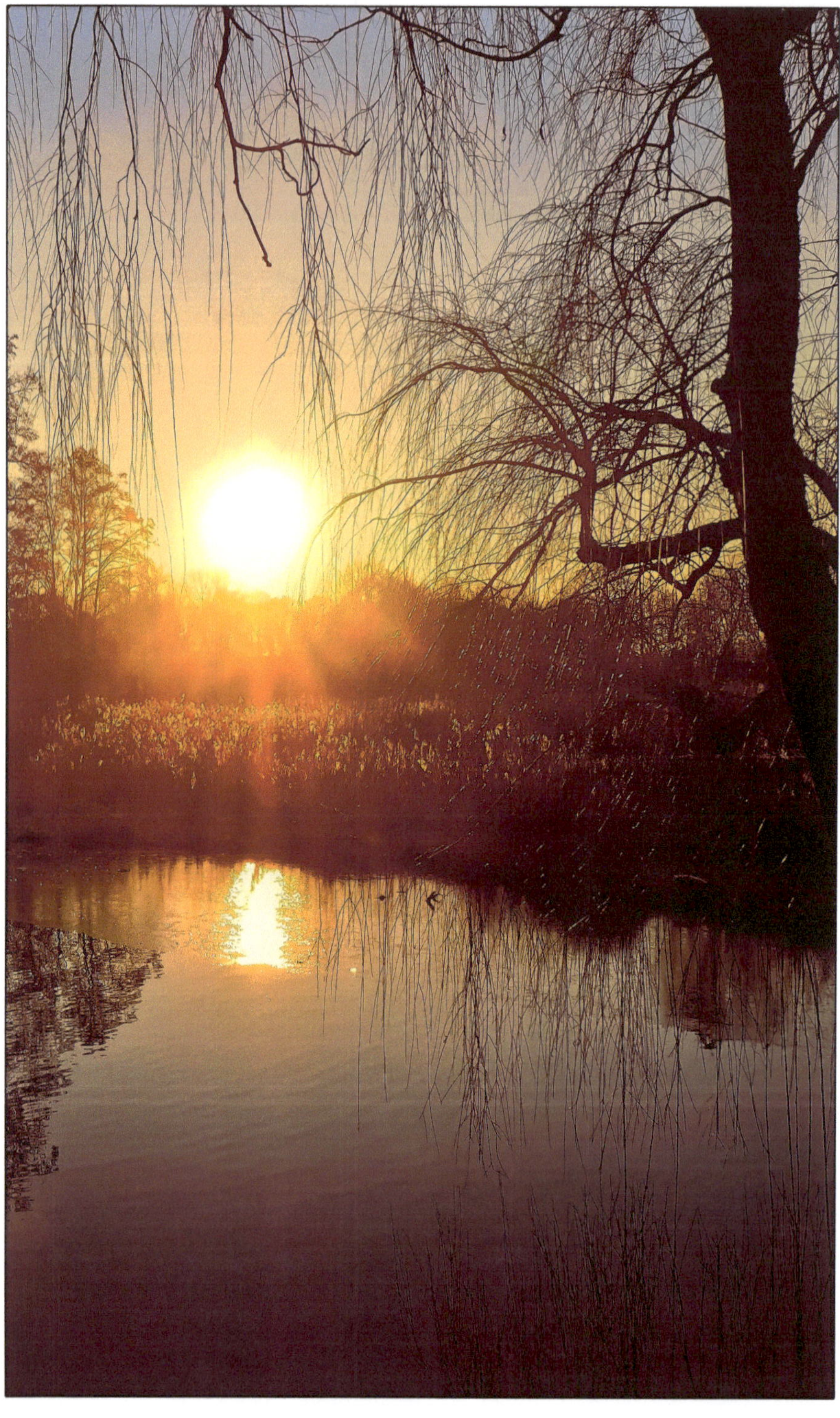

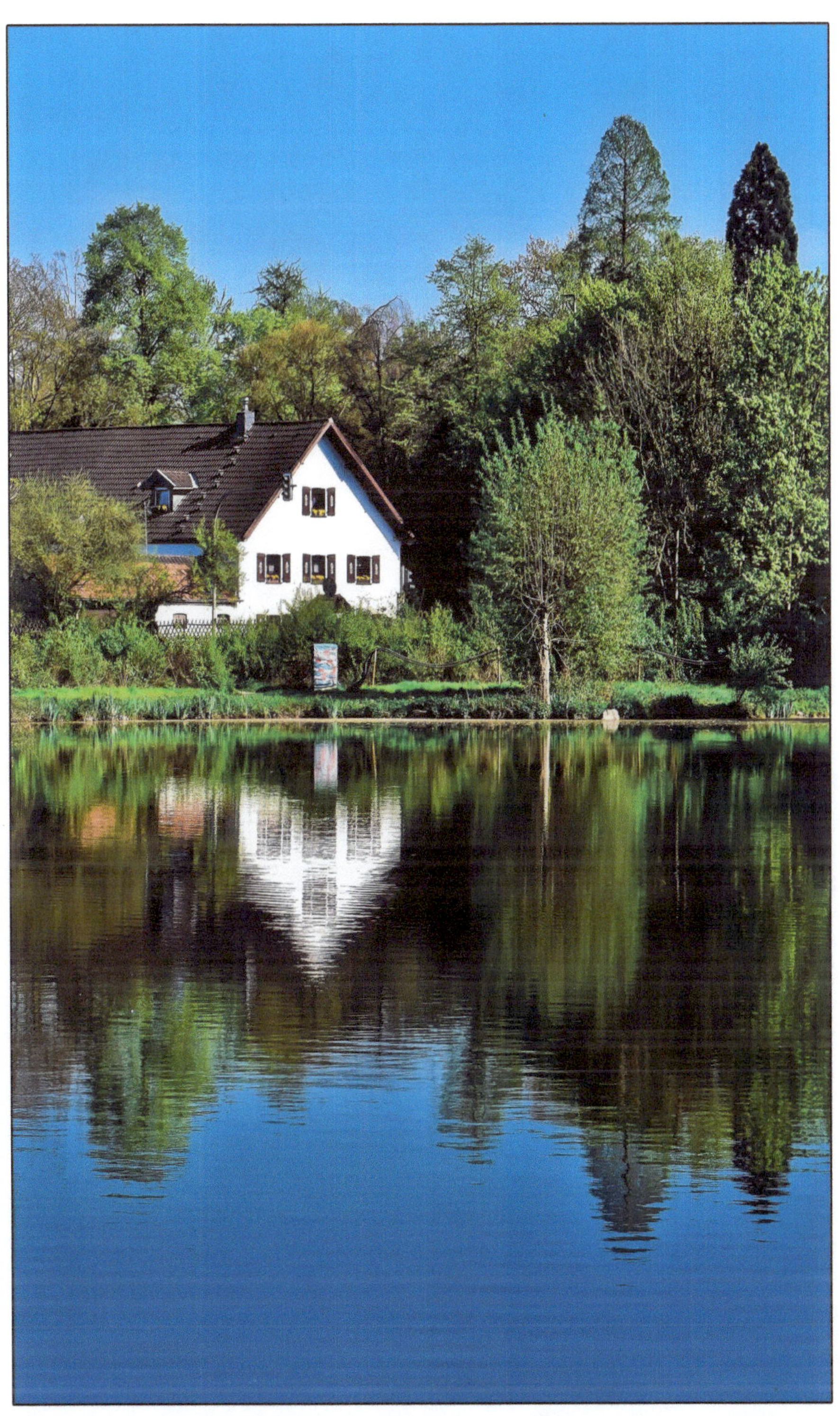

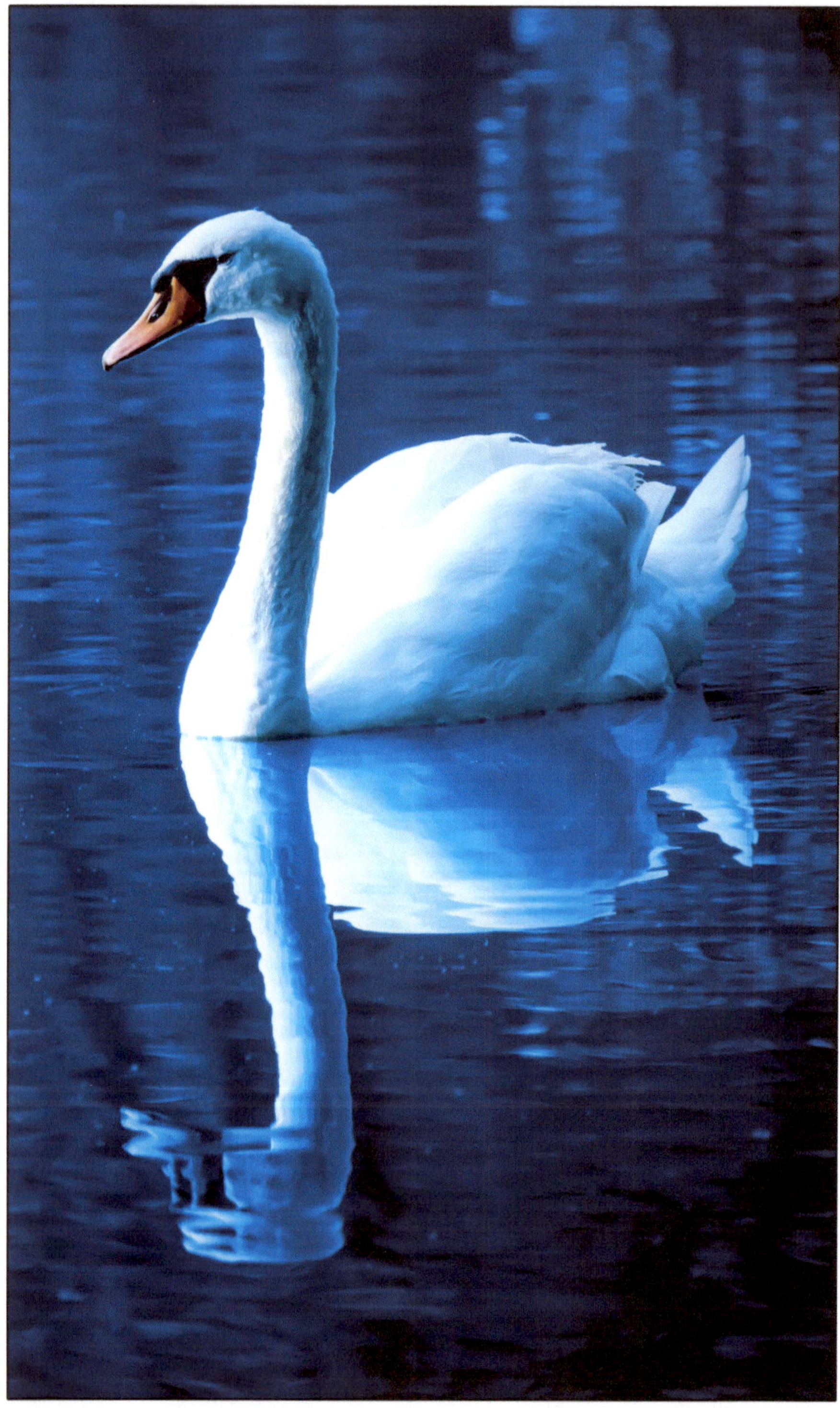

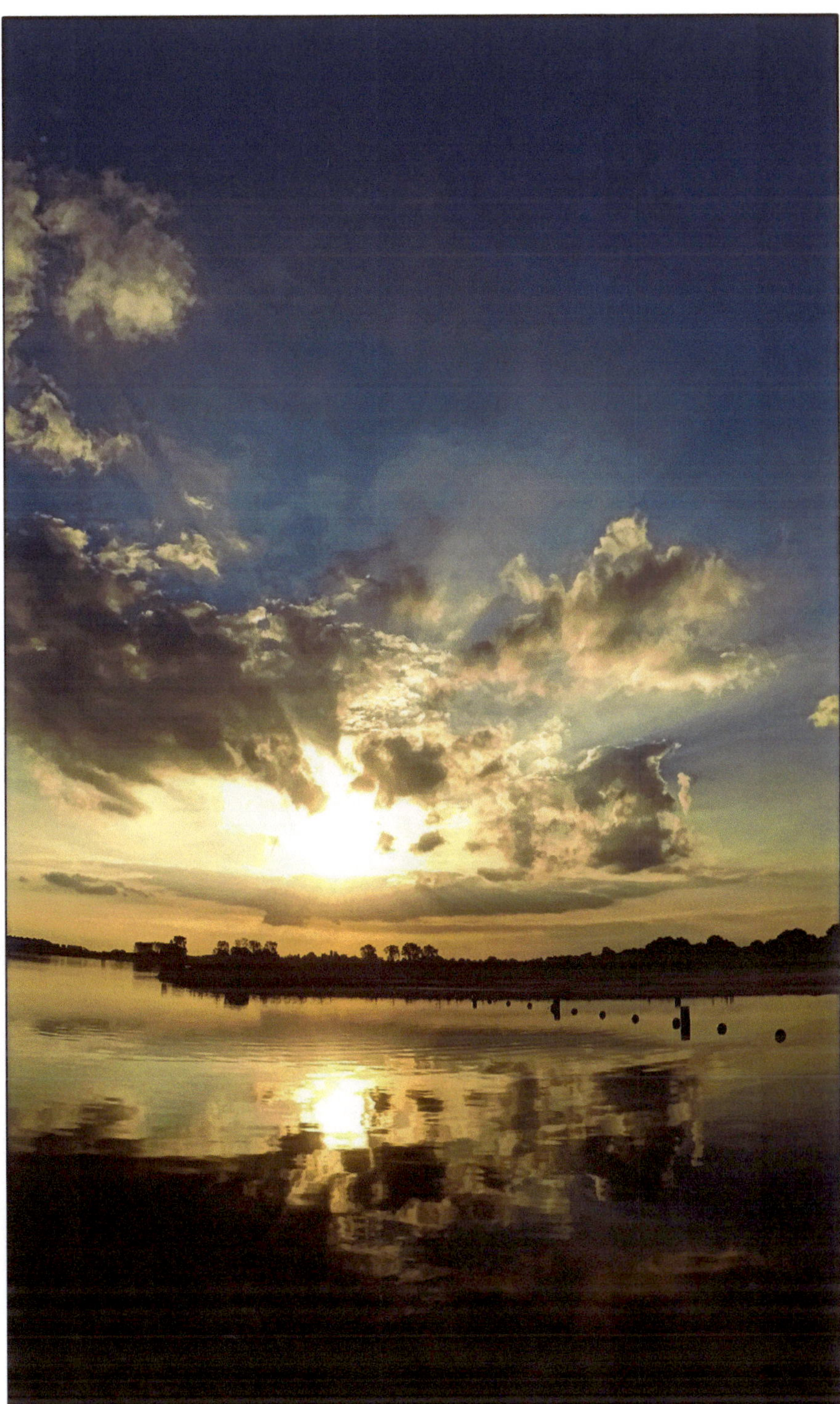

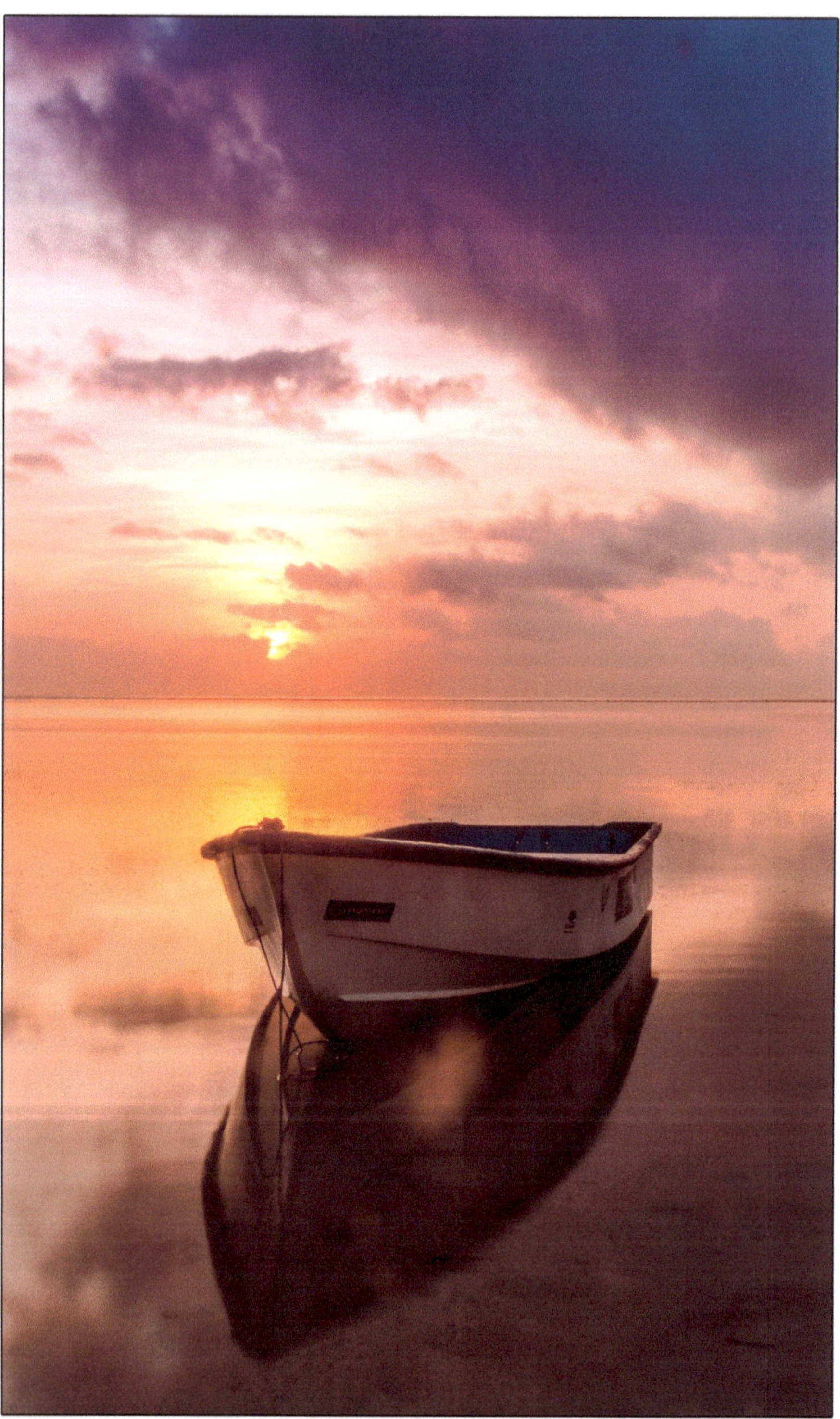

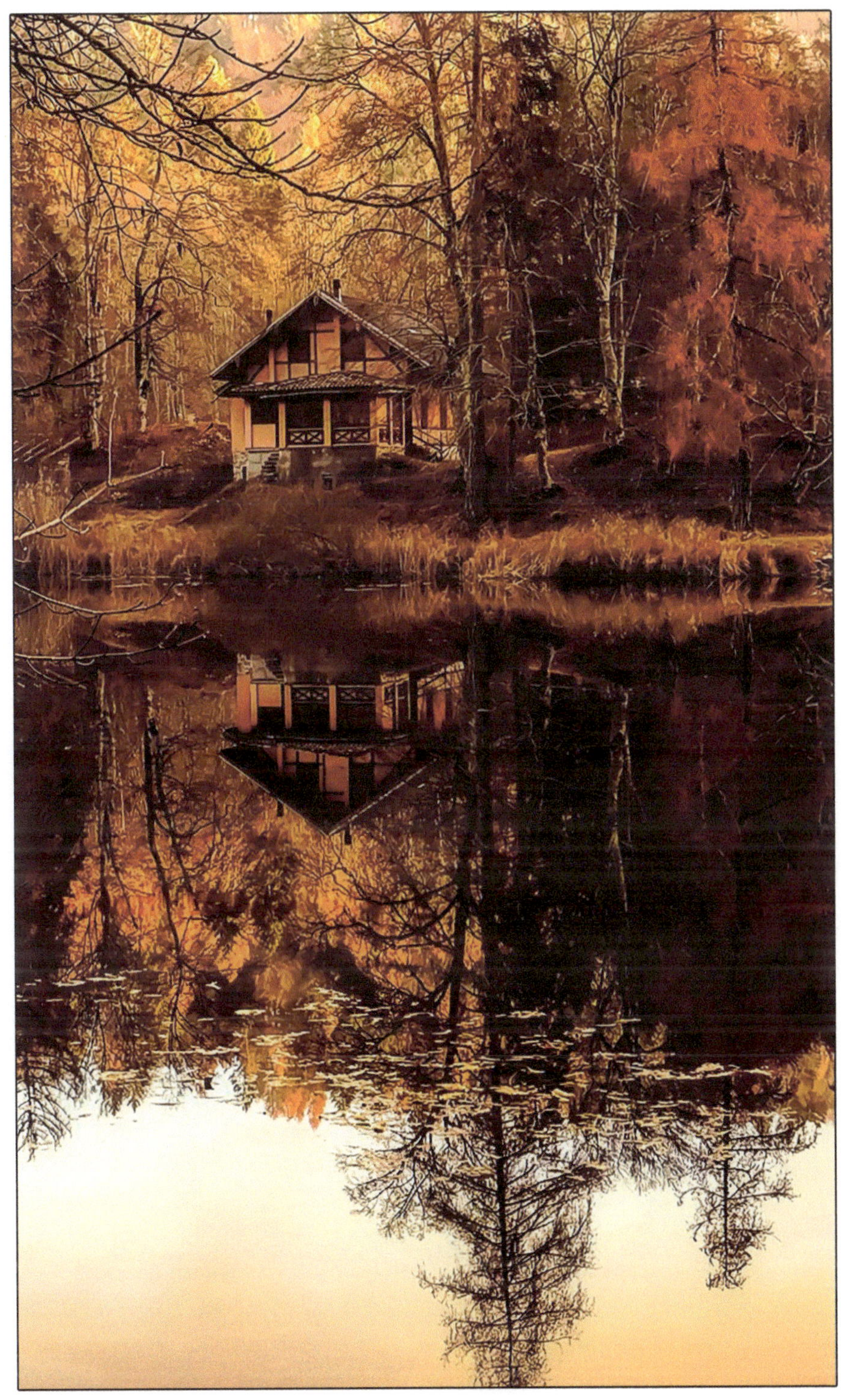

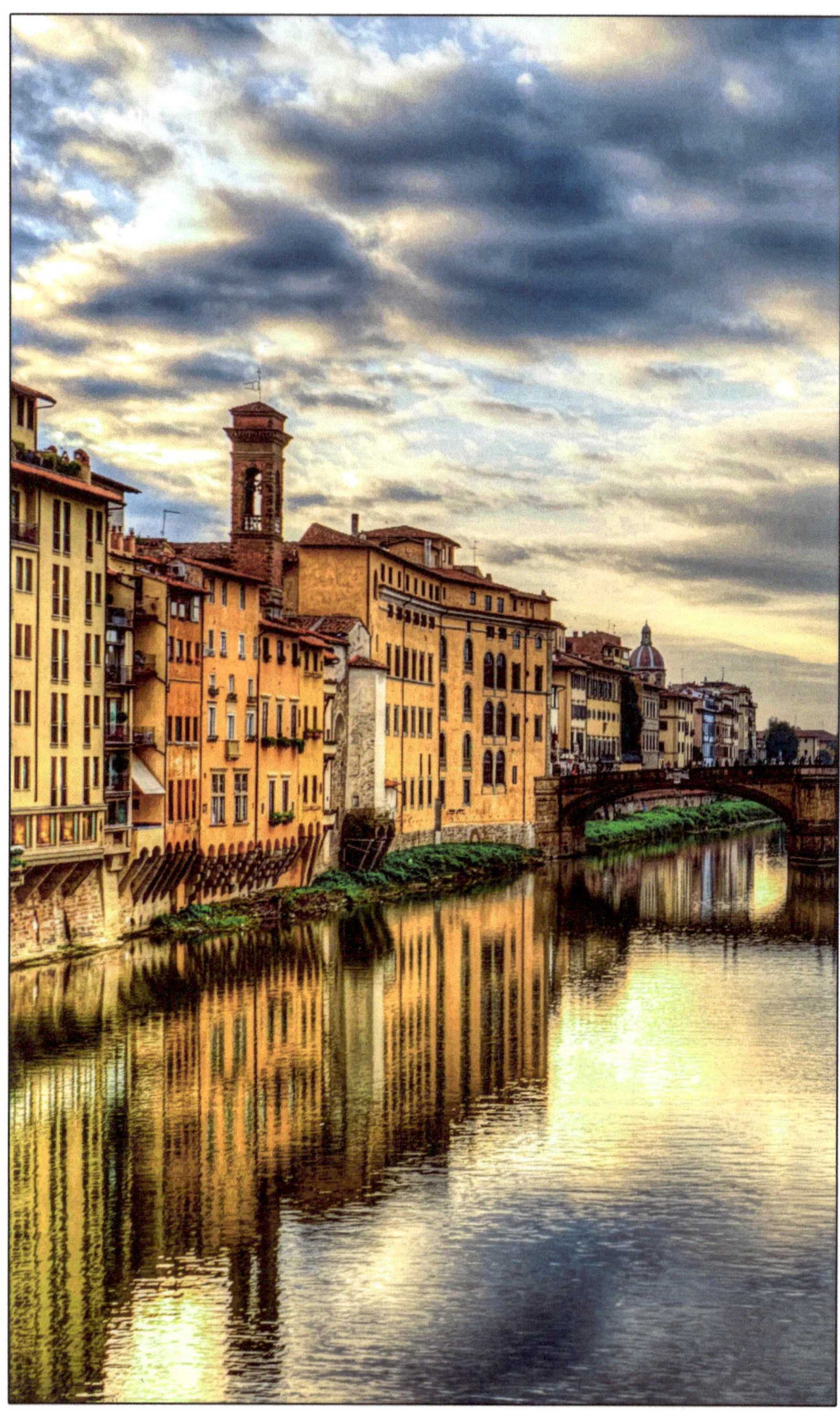

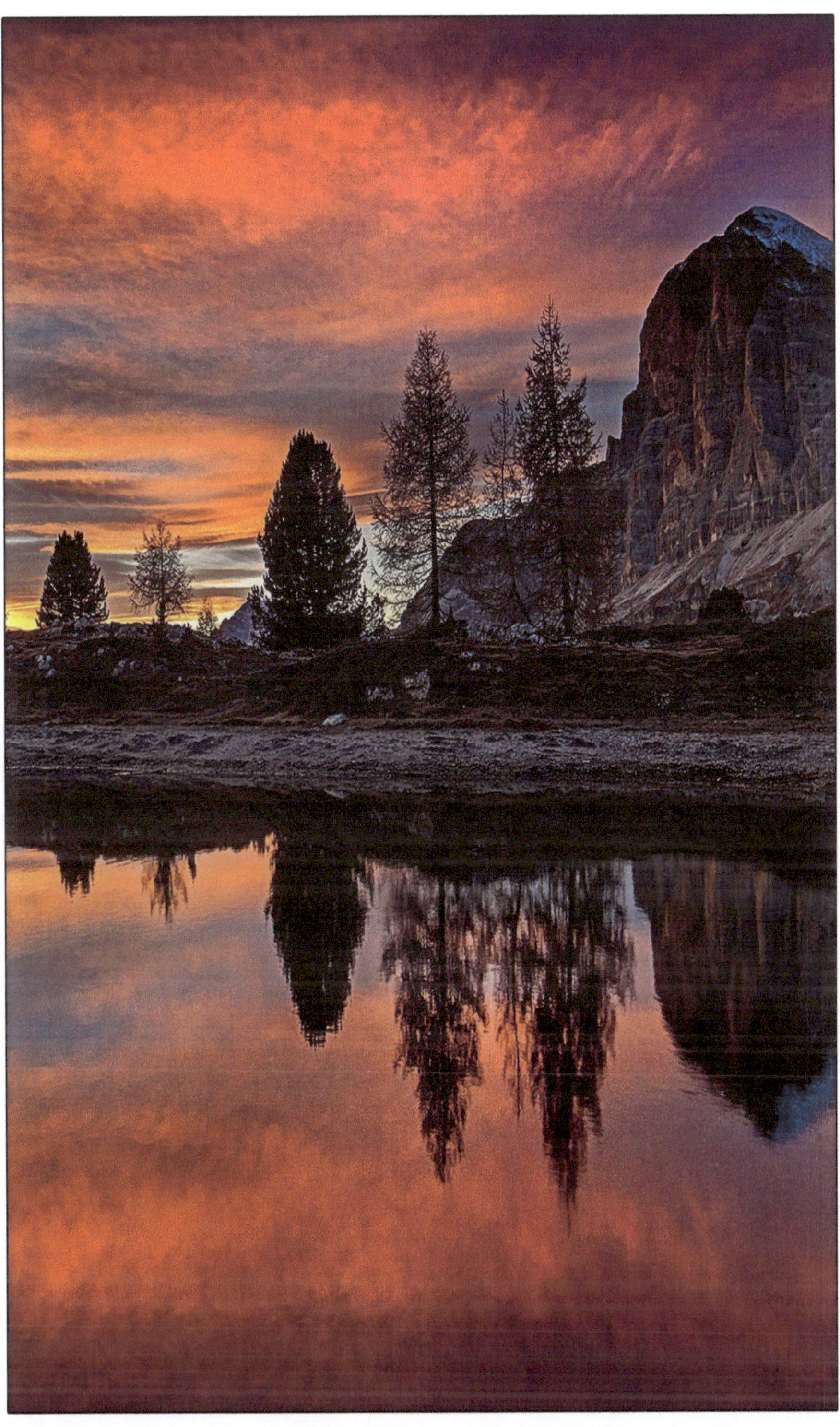

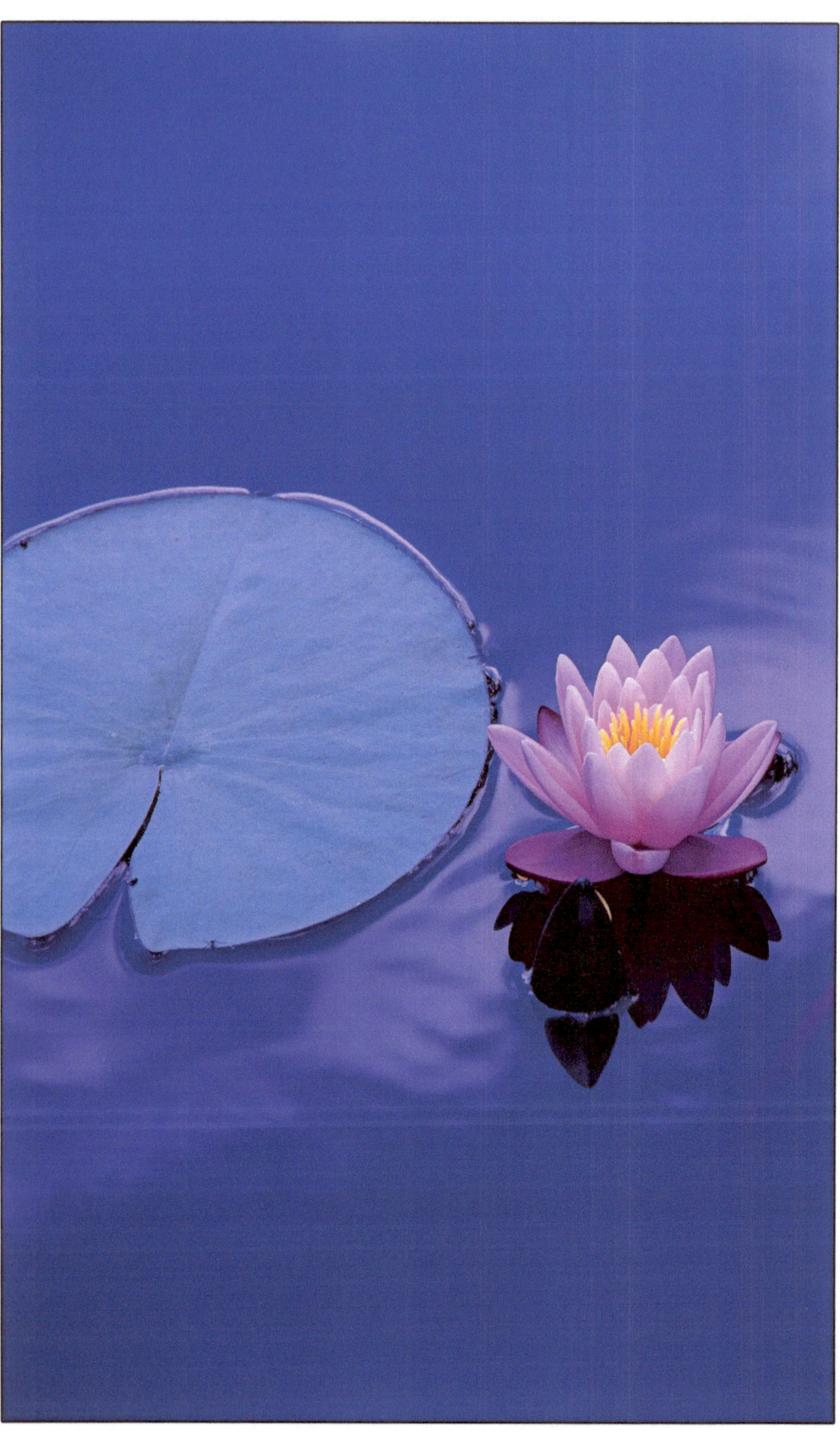

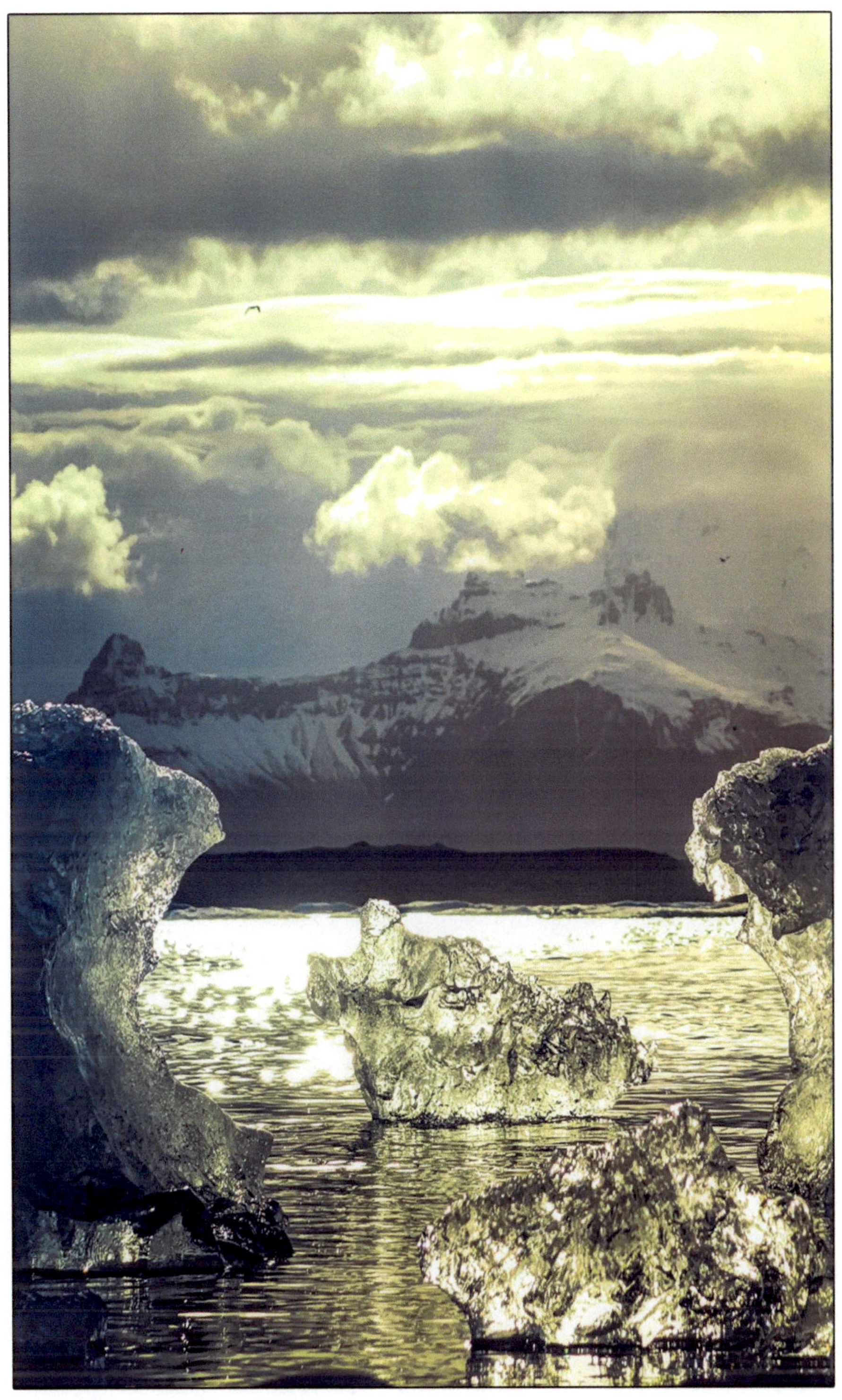

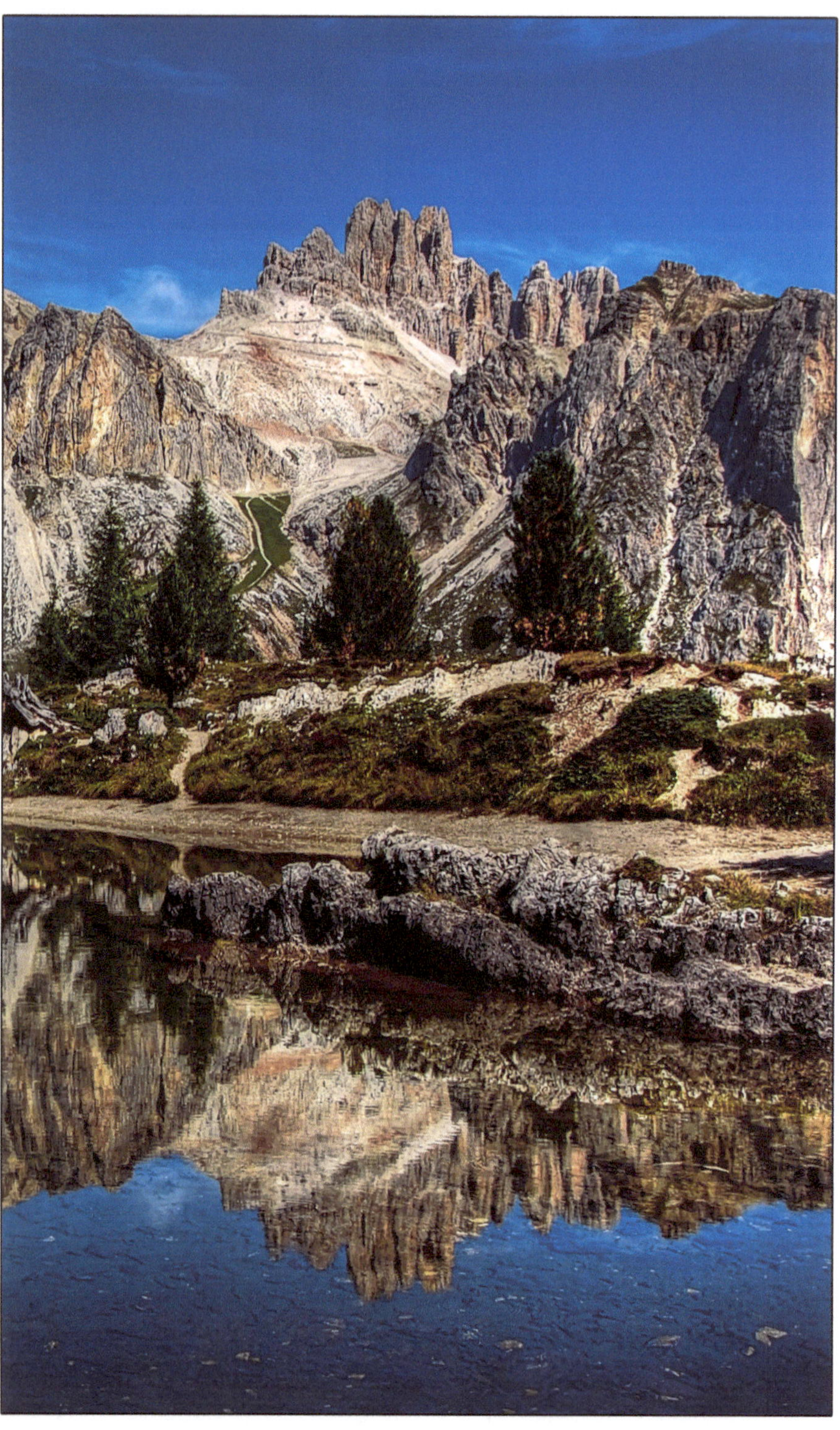

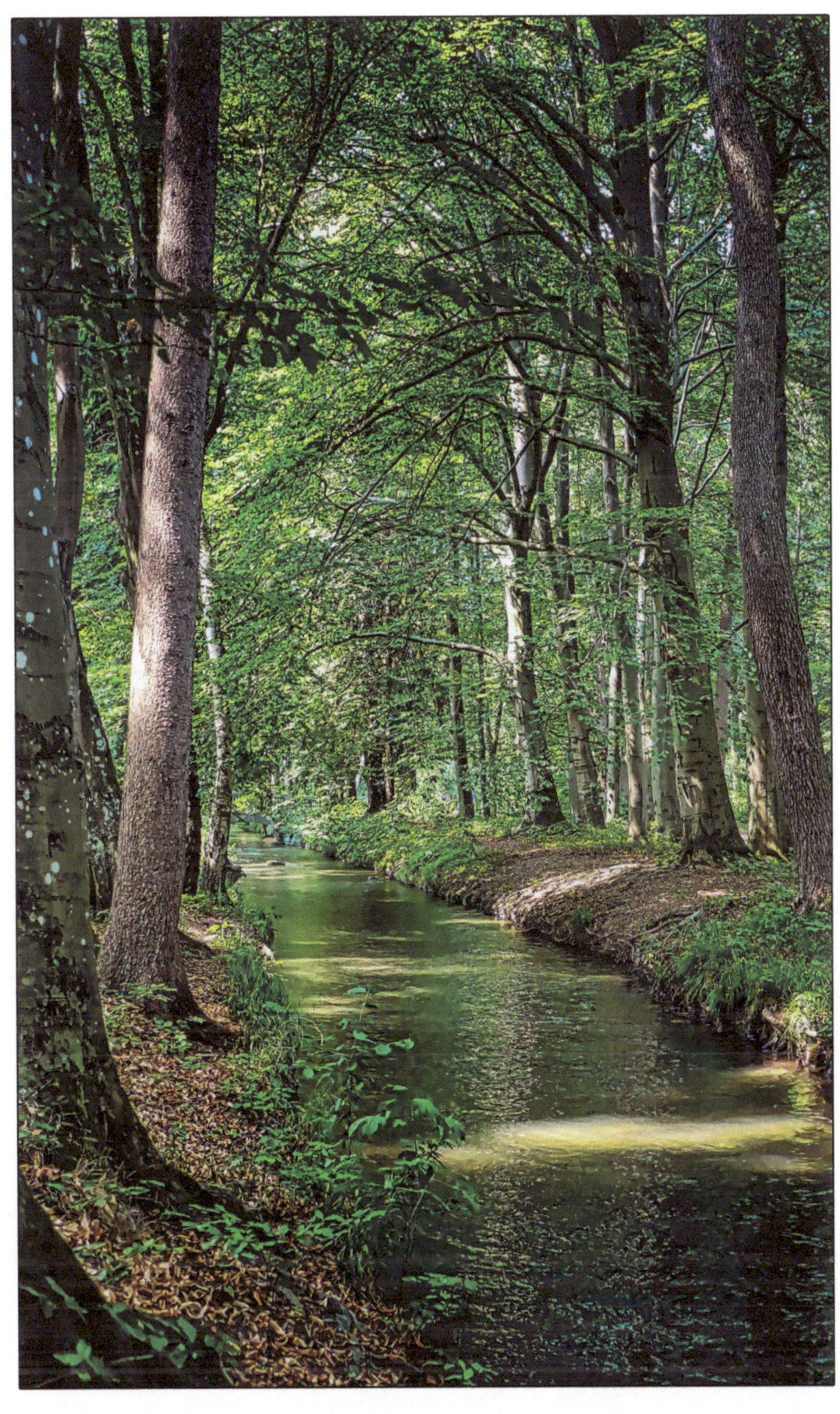

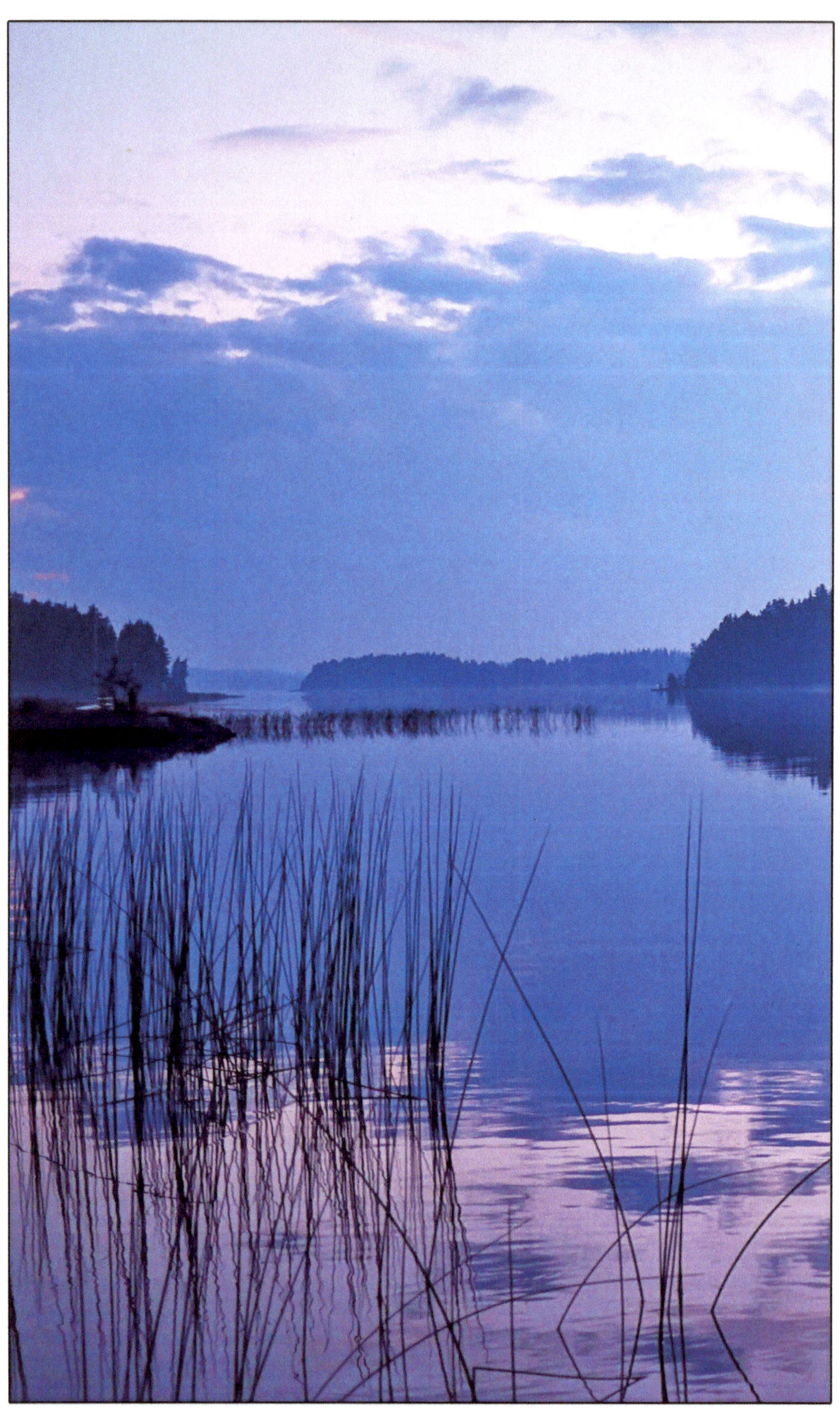

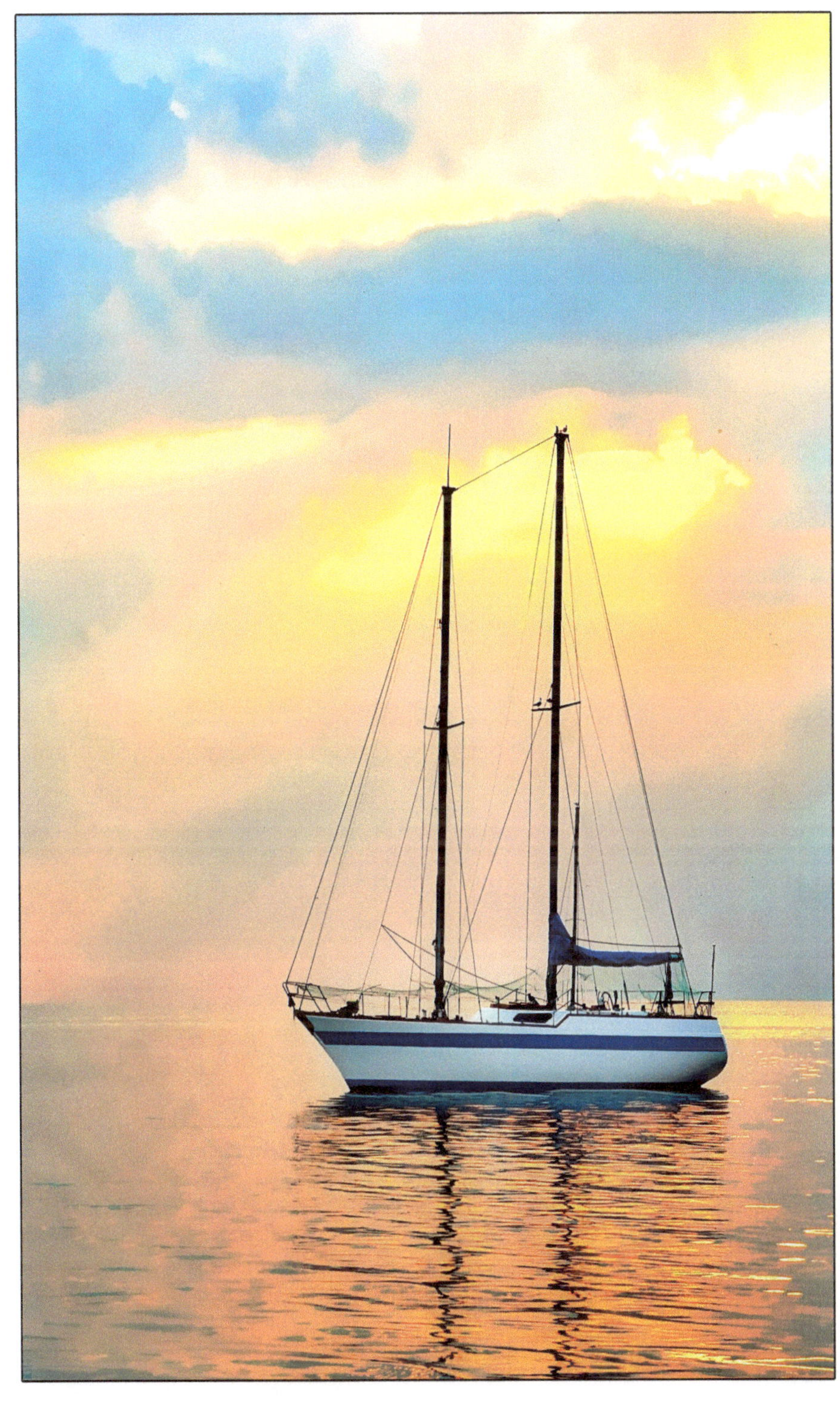

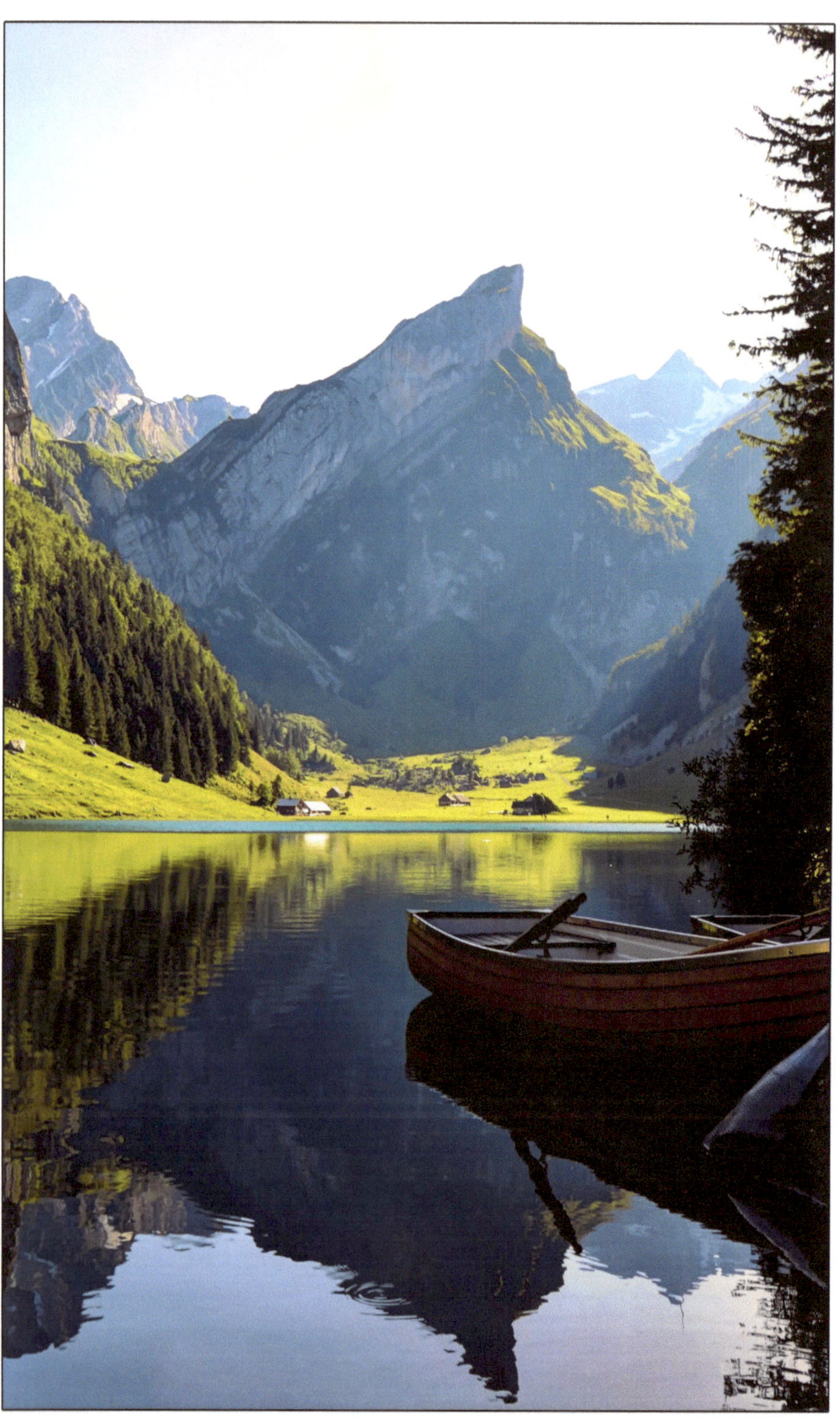

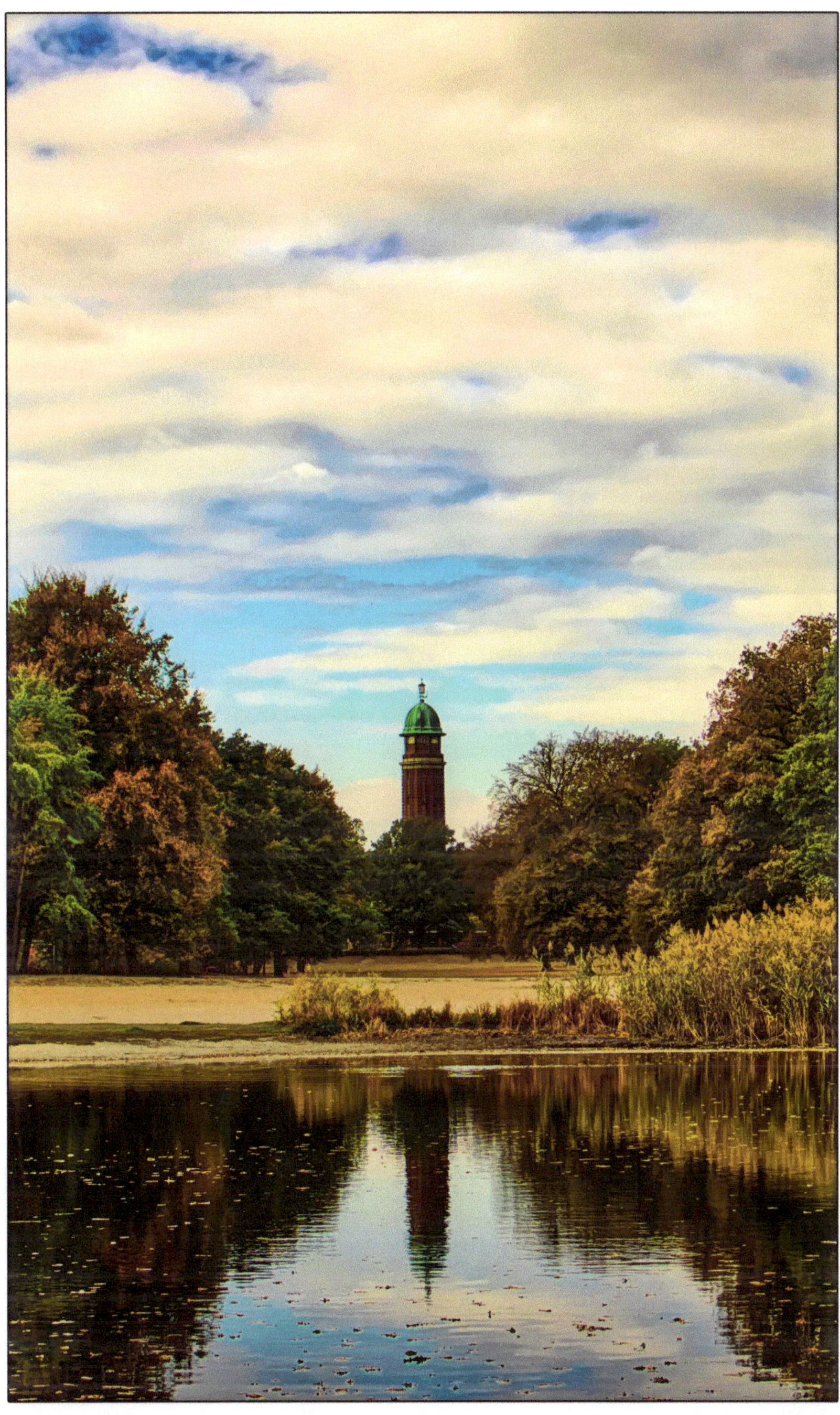

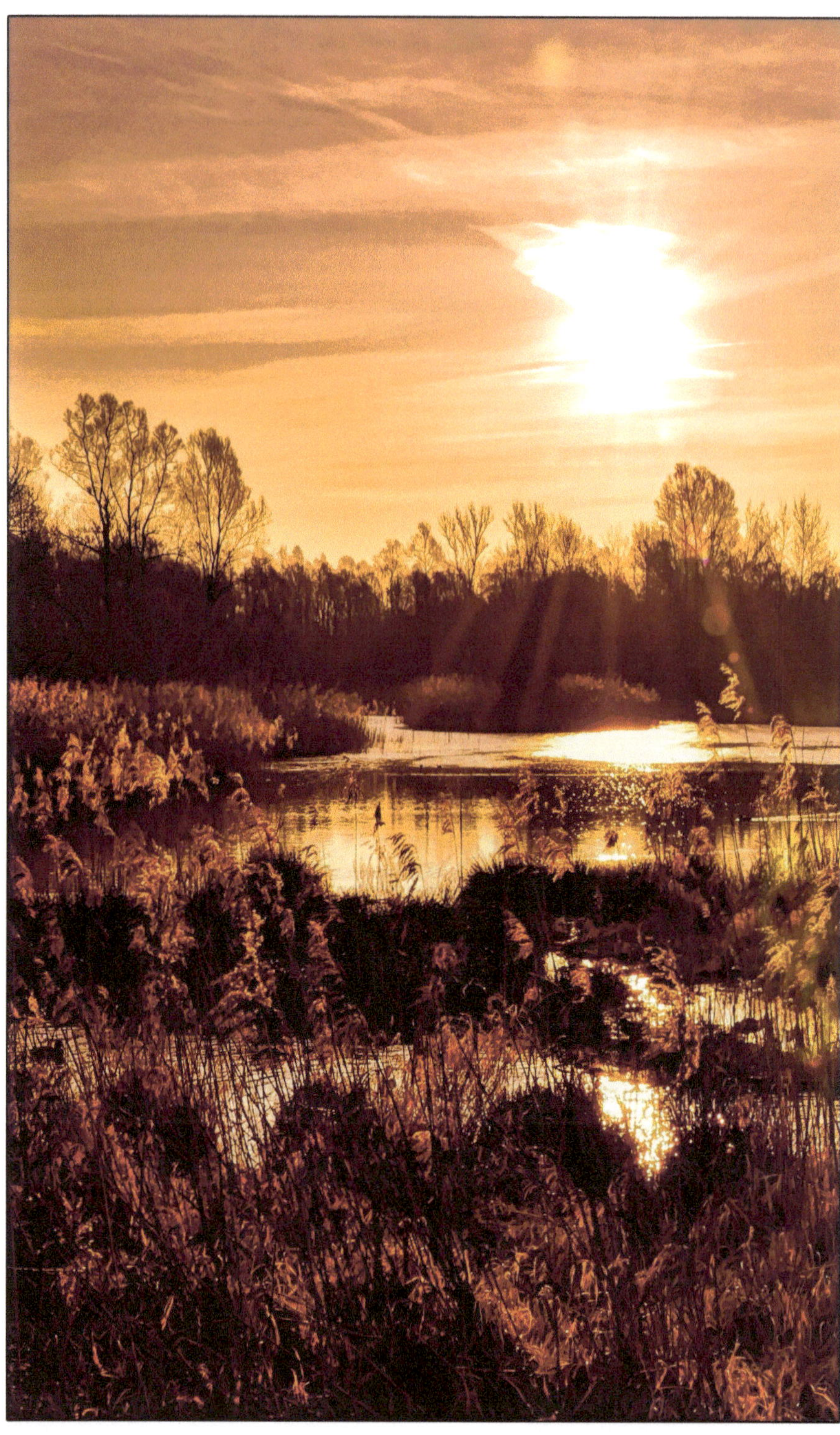

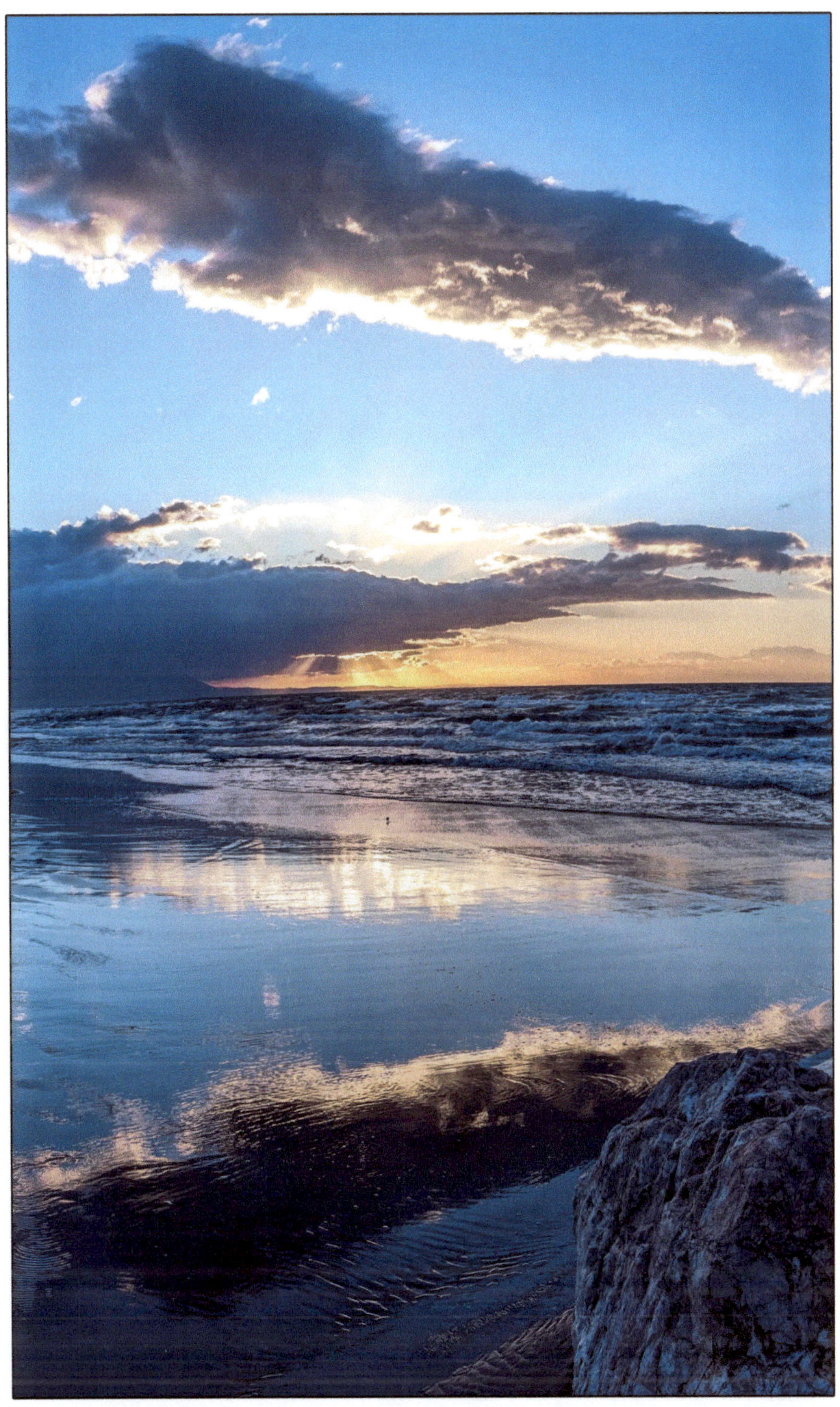

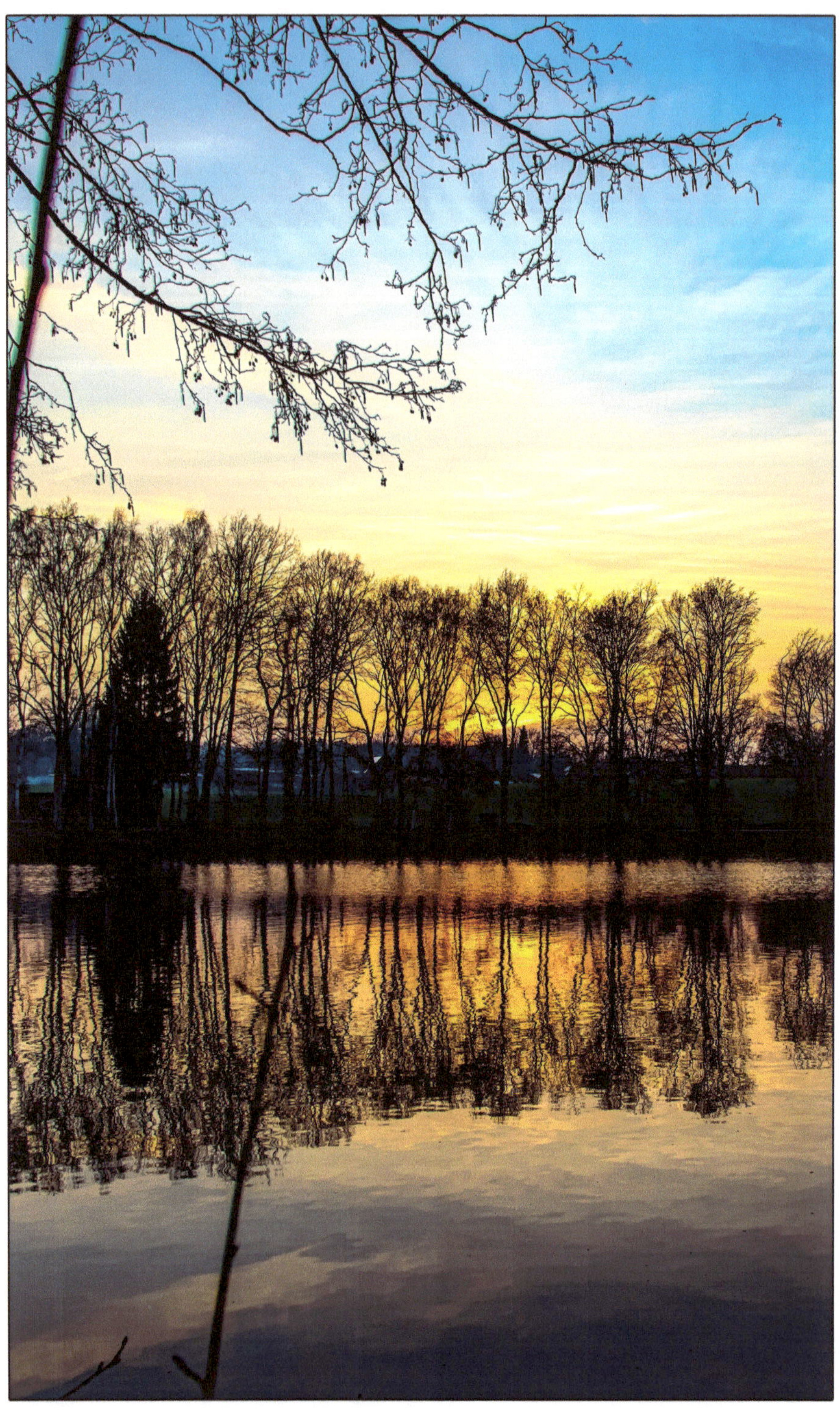

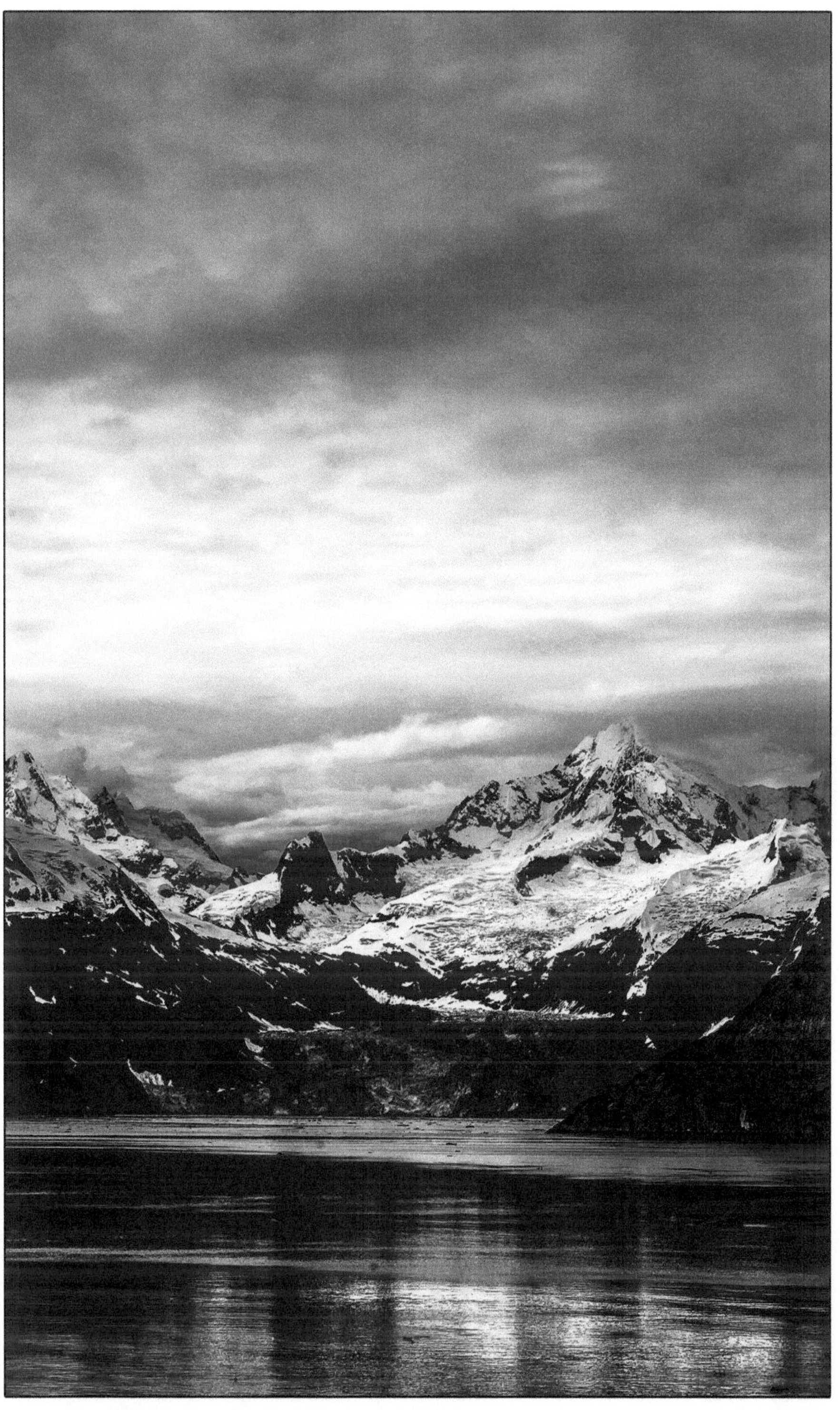

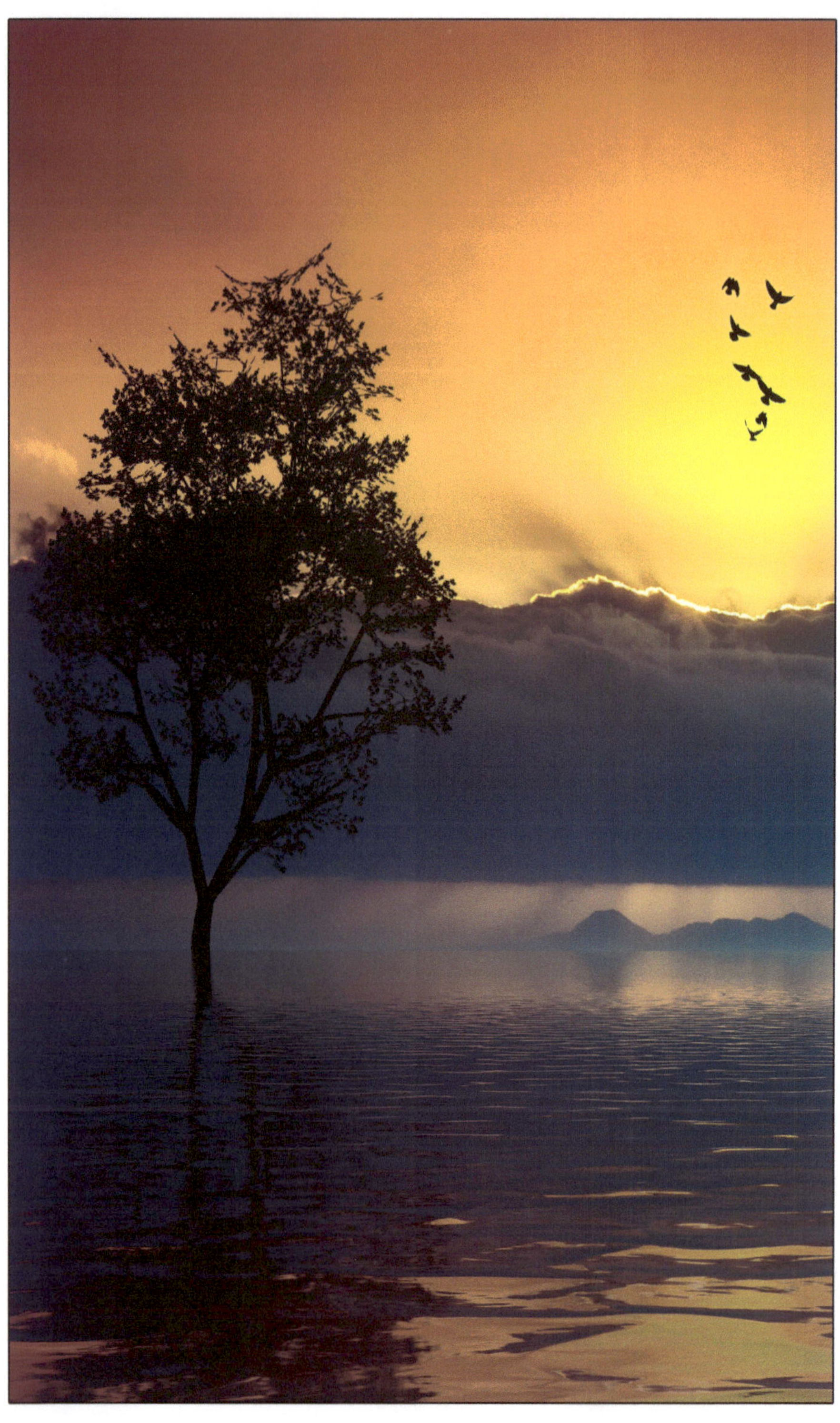

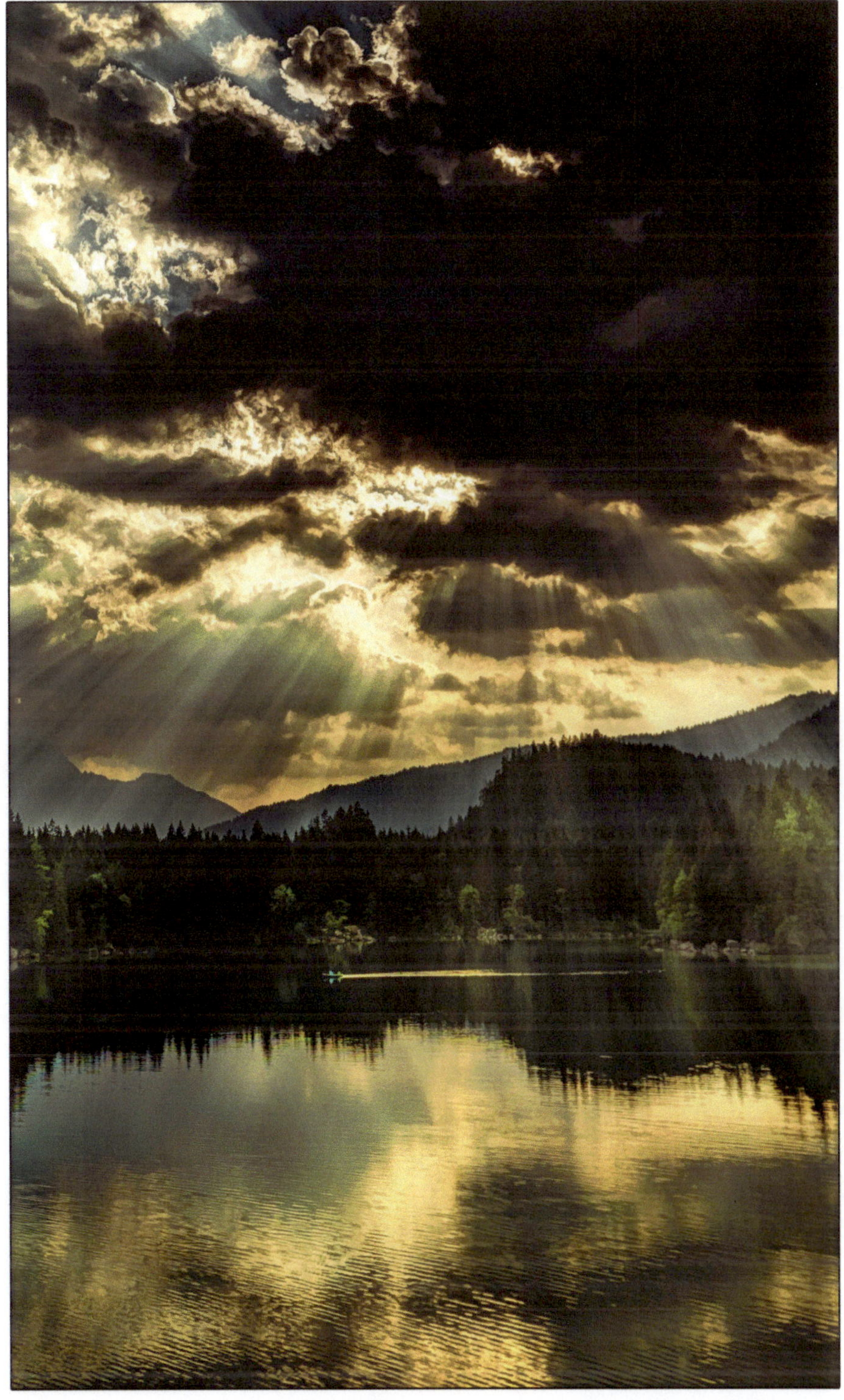

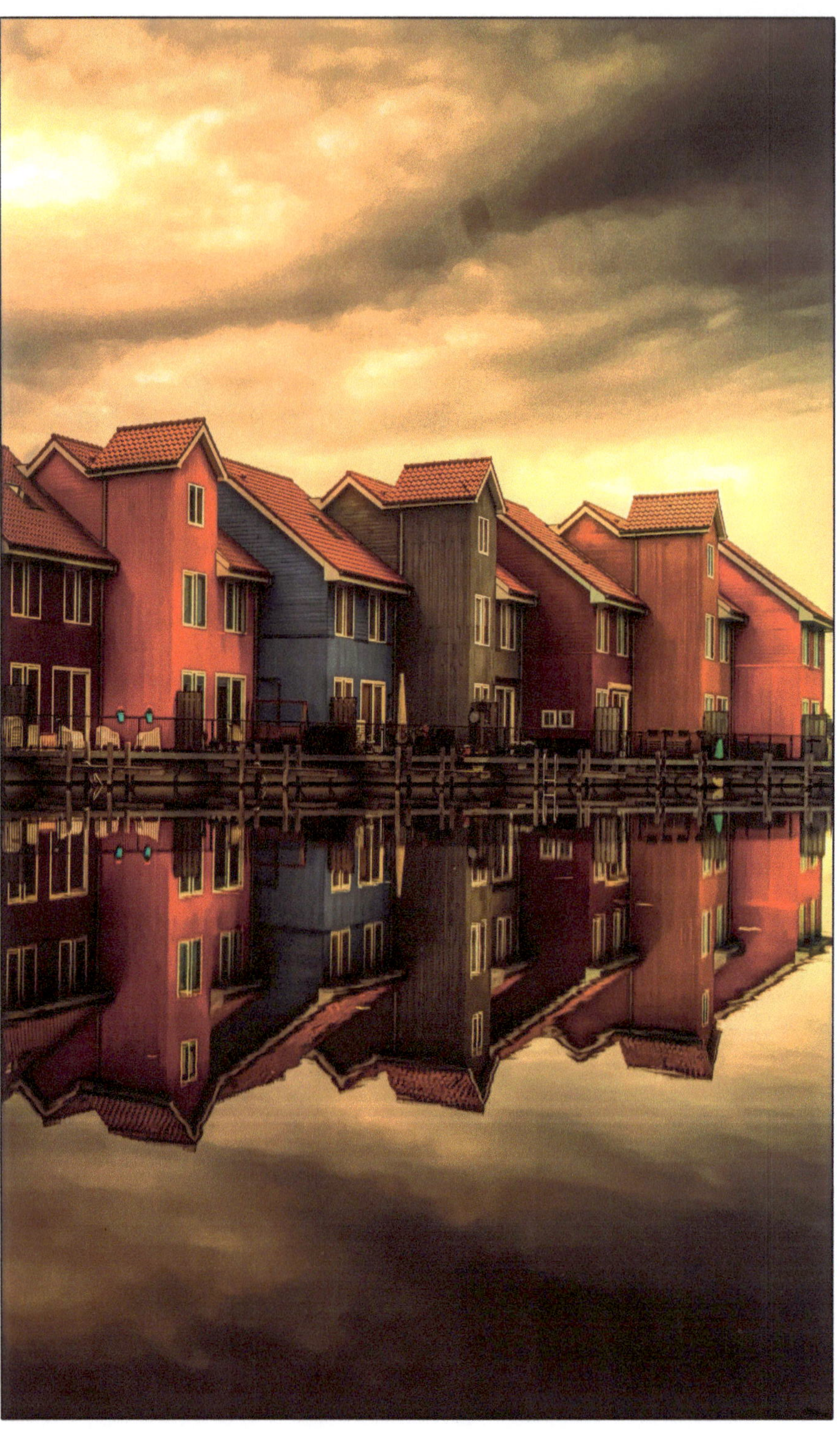

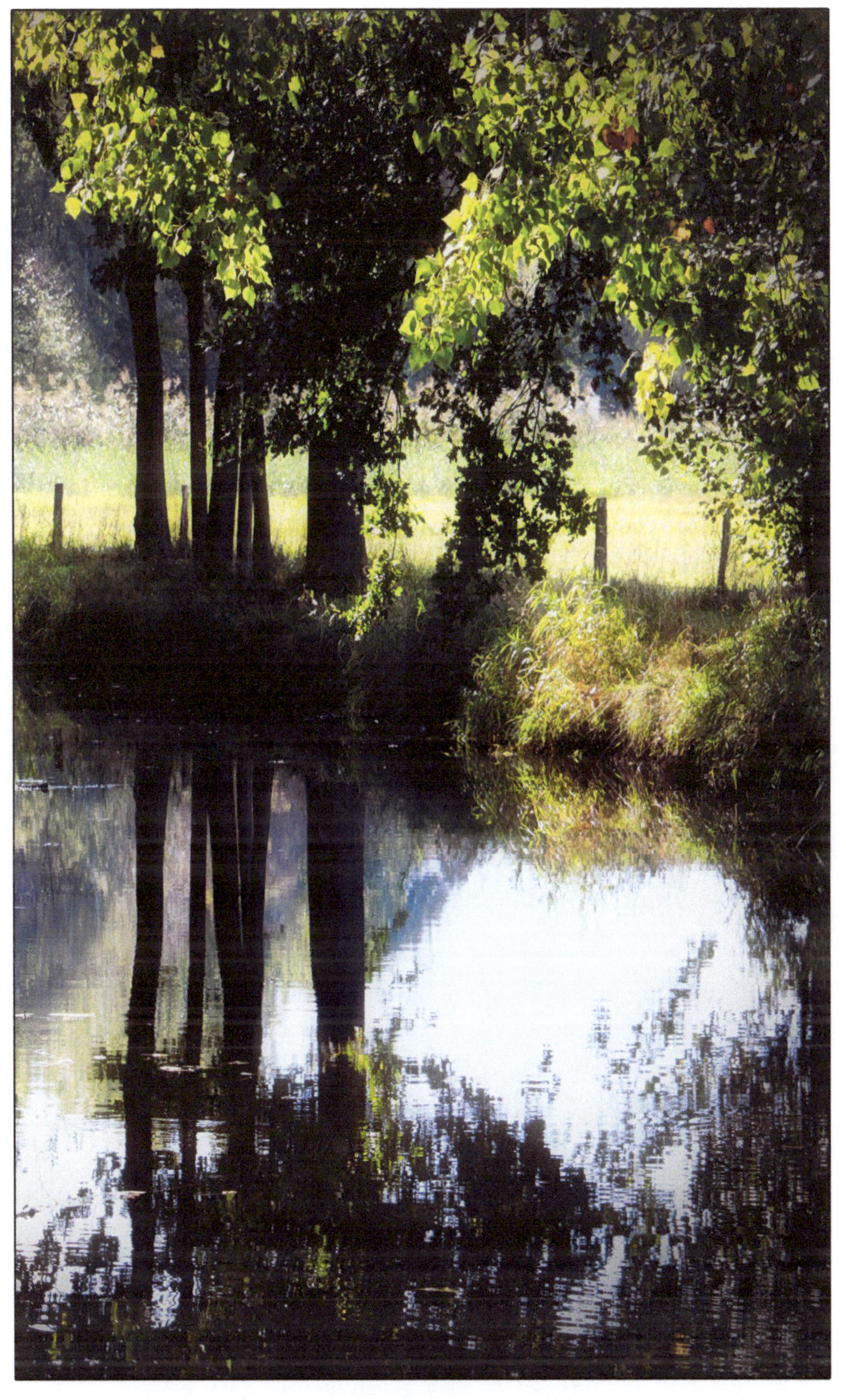

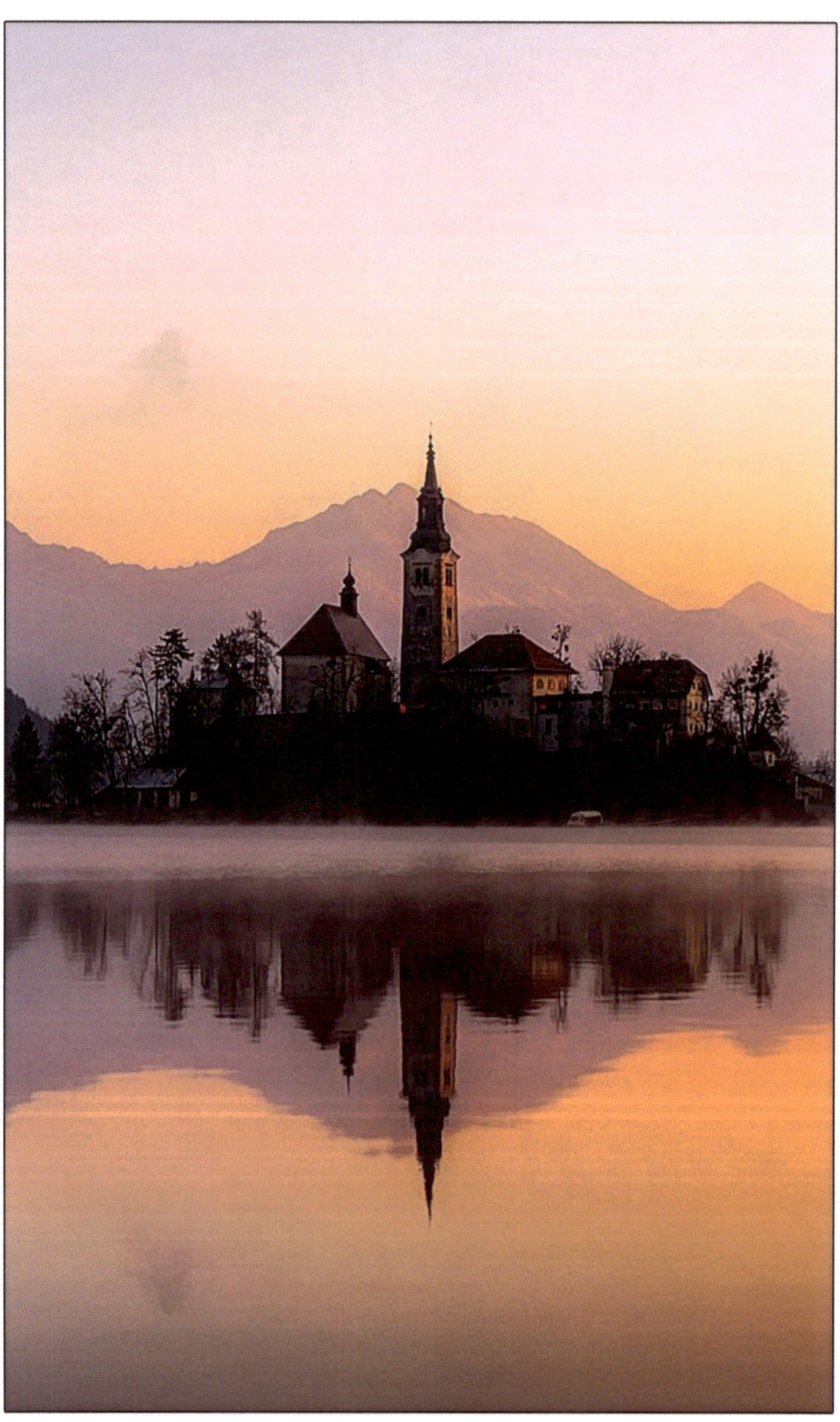

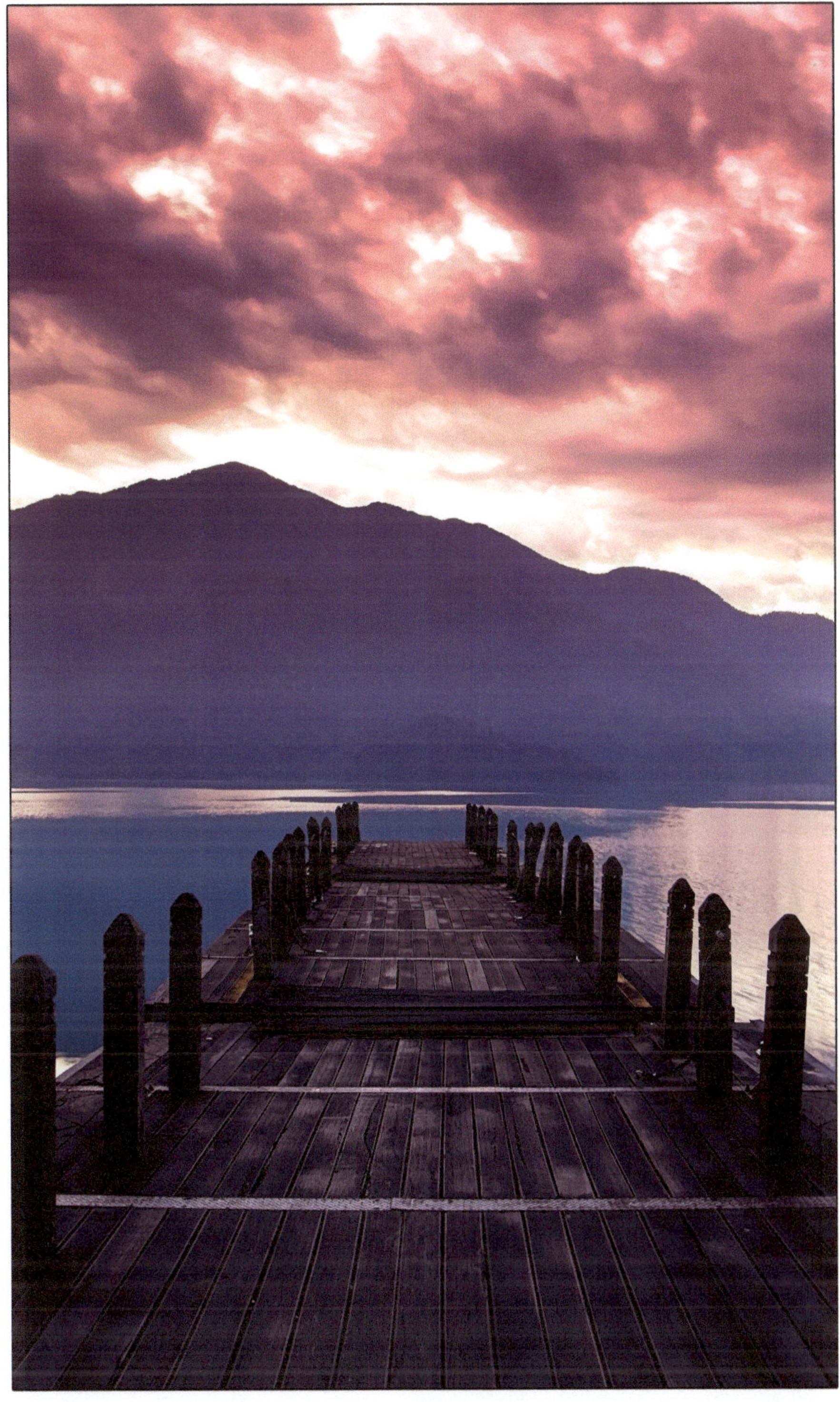